The Ketogenic Cookbook

Quick and Delicious Recipes to
Lose Weight With Ketogenic Diet

by

Susan L. Williams

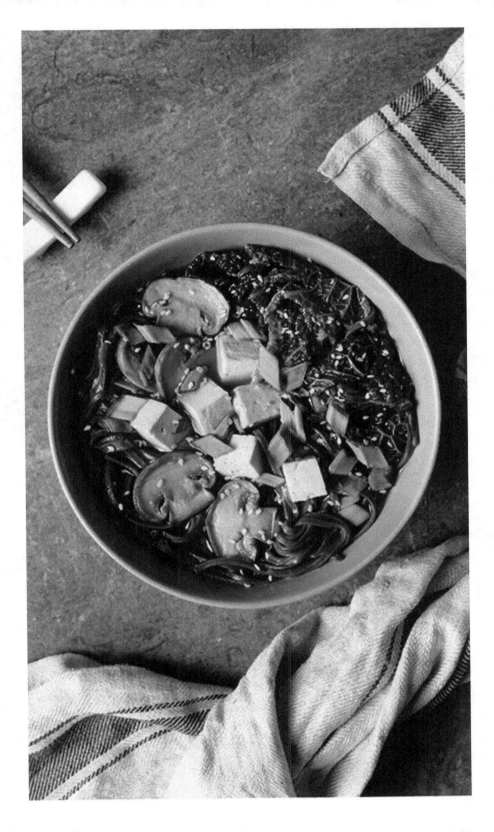

TABLE OF CONTENTS

TABLE OF CONTENTS

TABLE OF CONTENTS

Chicken Wings

2/3 cup butter | 1/4 cup Dijon-style prepared mustard

1 1/4 cups dried bread crumbs, seasoned | 1/4 cup Parmesan cheese

20 chicken wings, tips discarded

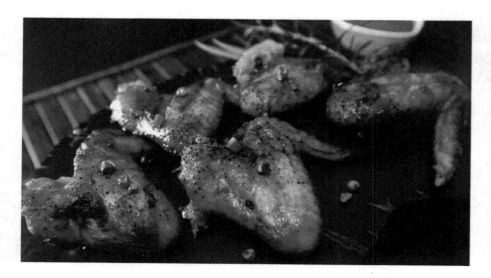

Directions:

Preheat oven to 400 degrees F (205 degrees C).

Melt butter or margarine and stir in mustard.

Place bread crumbs in a flat dish.

Roll each chicken piece in the butter mixture,

then coat with bread crumbs.

Place chicken pieces in a 9x13 inch baking dish.

Sprinkle with cheese and bake in the p

reheated oven for 15 minutes.

Turn and bake 15 minutes longer, or until crispy.

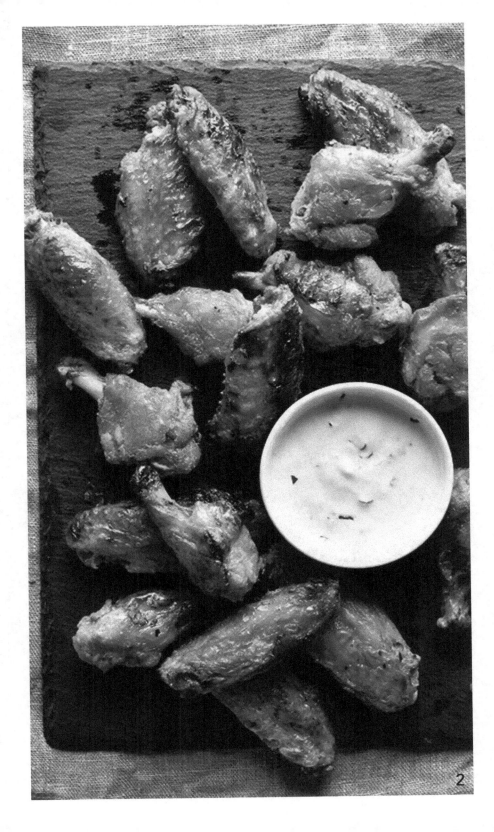

Fruited Chicken

1 large onion, sliced | 6 boneless, skinless chicken breast halves

1/3 cup orange juice | 2 tablespoons soy sauce

2 tablespoons Worcestershire sauce | 2 tablespoons Dijon mustard

1 tablespoon grated orange peel | 2 garlic cloves, minced

1/2 cup chopped dried apricots | 1/2 cup dried cranberries hot cooked rice

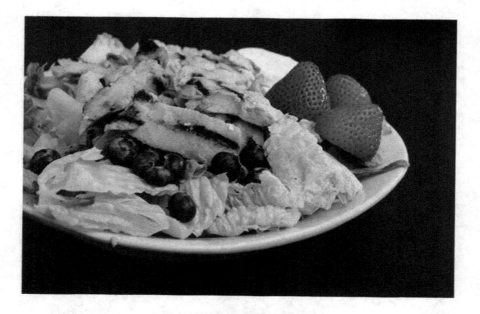

Directions:

Place onion and chicken in a 5-qt. slow cooker.
Combine the orange juice, soy sauce,
Worcestershire sauce, mustard, orange peel and garlic; pour over chicken.
Sprinkle with apricots and cranberries.
Cover and cook on low for 7-8 hours or until chicken juices run clear.
Serve over rice.

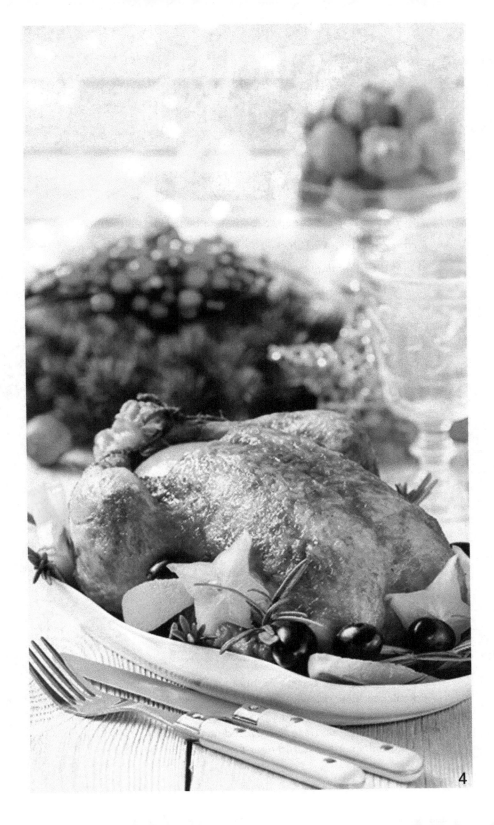

4

Chicken Brunch Bake

Ingredients:

9 slices day-old bread, cubed | 3 cups chicken broth

4 cups cubed cooked chicken | 1/2 cup uncooked instant rice

1 cup diced pimientos | 2 tablespoons minced fresh parsley

1 1/2 teaspoons salt (optional) | 4 eggs, beaten

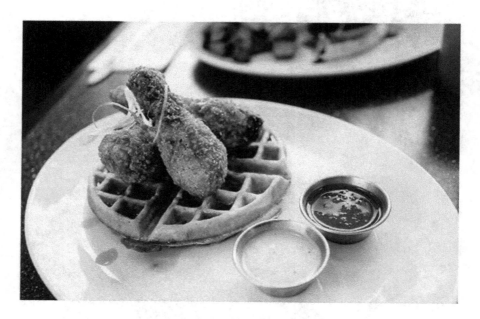

Directions:

In a large bowl, toss bread cubes and broth.
Add chicken, rice, pimientos, parsley and salt if desired; mix well.
Transfer to a greased 13-in. x 9-in. x 2-in. baking dish.
Pour eggs over all. Bake, uncovered, at 325 degrees for 1 hour
or until a knife inserted near the center comes out clean.

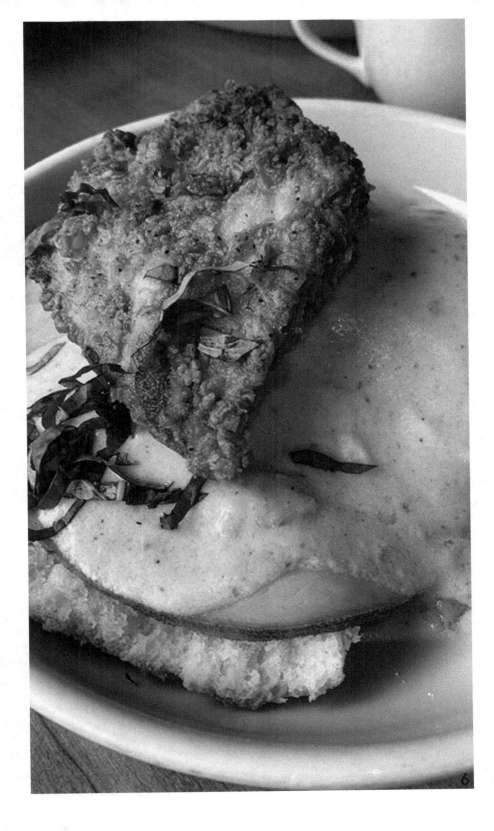

6

Southwestern Chicken

2 teaspoons garlic powder | 1 teaspoon chili powder

1/2 teaspoon salt | 1/2 teaspoon paprika

4 (4 ounce) boneless, skinless chicken breast halves

2 teaspoons lime juice

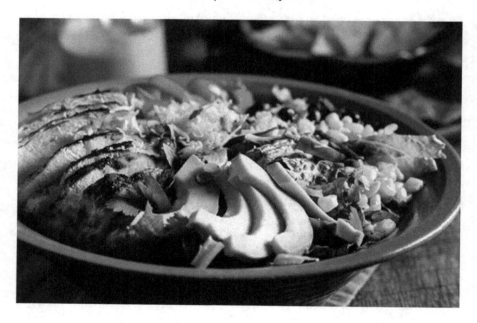

Directions:

In a small bowl, combine the garlic powder, chili powder,
salt and paprika. Rub over both sides of chicken.
In a large skillet coated with nonstick cooking spray,
brown chicken on both sides;
drizzle with lime juice.
Cover and cook for 5-7 minutes or until chicken juices run clear.

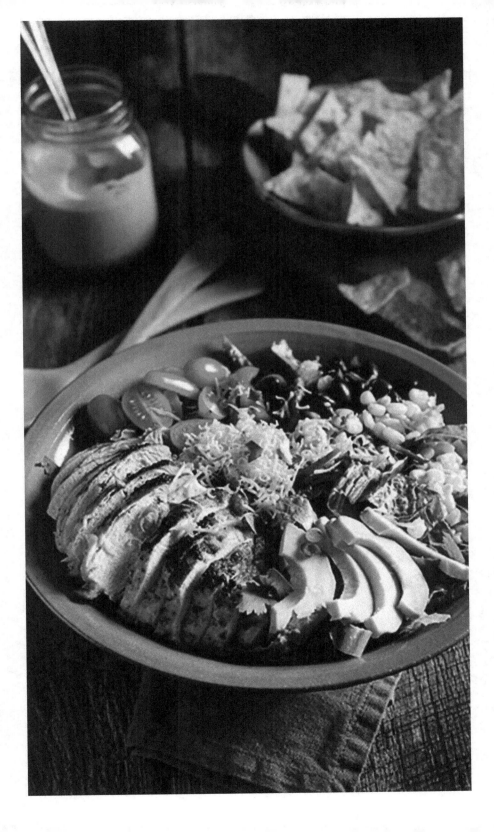

Delicious Baked Chicken

4 bone-in chicken breast halves, with skin | 1 tablespoon olive oil

1 pinch garlic powder | salt and pepper to taste

3/4 cup Worcestershire sauce

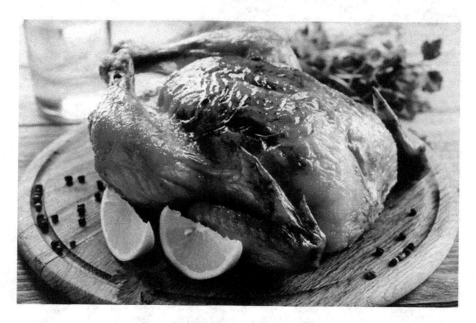

Directions:

Preheat oven to 350 degrees F (175 degrees C).
Rub each chicken breast with olive oil,
then place in a lightly greased 9x13 inch baking dish.
Season with garlic powder, salt and pepper to taste.
Pour Worcestershire sauce over each breast.
Cover dish with aluminum foil and bake in the
preheated oven for 45 minutes.
Check chicken and remove cover if desired.
Bake for another 15 minutes.

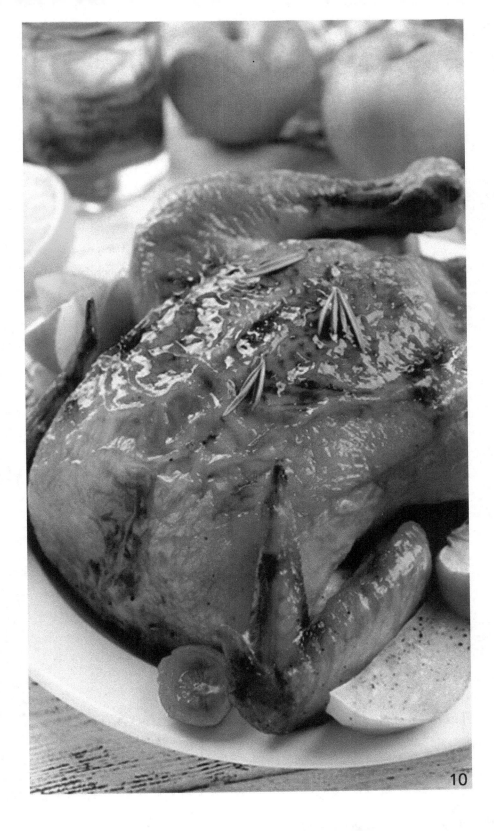

Oven Baked Herb Chicken

6 skinless, boneless chicken breasts

1 (1 ounce) package cheese and garlic dry salad dressing mix

2 tablespoons all-purpose flour | 1/4 teaspoon salt

1/4 cup butter | 1 tablespoon lemon juice

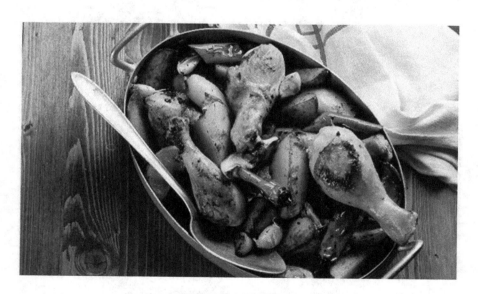

Directions:

Preheat oven to 350 degrees F (175 degrees C).
Place chicken in a lightly greased 9x13 inch baking dish.
In a small bowl, combine the dry salad dressing mix,
flour, salt, butter or margarine and lemon juice.
Mix together, then brush mixture evenly over the top of the chicken breasts.
Bake in the preheated oven for 60 minutes or until tender.

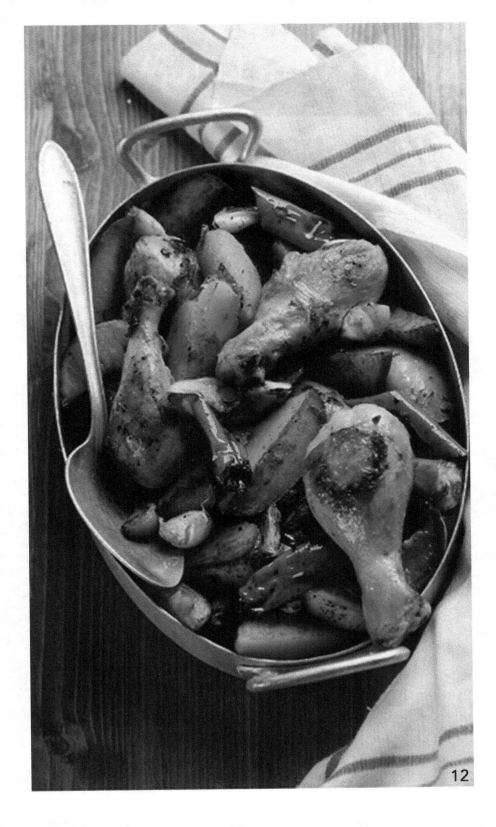

12

BBQ Chicken Wings

Ingredients:

1/2 cup teriyaki sauce | 1 cup oyster sauce

1/4 cup soy sauce | 1/4 cup ketchup

2 tablespoons garlic powder | 1/4 cup gin

2 dashes liquid smoke flavoring | 1/2 cup white sugar

1 1/2 pounds chicken wings, separated at joints, tips discarded

1/4 cup honey

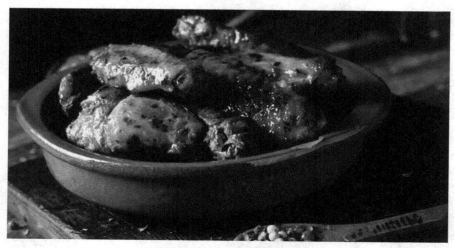

Directions:

In a large bowl, mix the teriyaki sauce, oyster sauce, soy sauce,
ketchup, garlic powder, gin, liquid smoke, and sugar.
Place the chicken wings in the bowl, cover,
and marinate in the refrigerator 8 hours or overnight.
Preheat the grill for low heat.
Lightly oil the grill grate.
Arrange chicken on the grill, and discard the marinade.
Grill the chicken wings on one side for 20 minutes,
then turn and brush with honey.
Continue grilling 25 minutes, or until juices run clear.

13

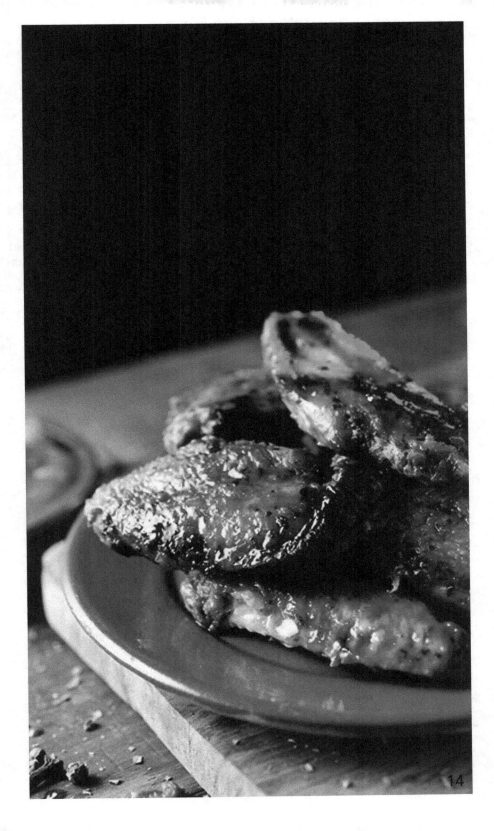

Restaurant-Style Buffalo Chicken Wings

Ingredients:

oil for deep frying

1/4 cup butter

1/4 cup hot sauce

1 dash ground black pepper

1 dash garlic powder

1/2 cup all-purpose flour

1/4 teaspoon paprika

1/4 teaspoon cayenne pepper

1/4 teaspoon salt 10 chicken wings

Directions:

Heat oil in a deep fryer to 375 degrees F (190 degrees C).
The oil should be just enough to cover wings entirely,
an inch or so deep. Combine the butter, hot sauce, pepper
and garlic powder in a small saucepan over low heat.
Stir together and heat until butter is melted and mixture is
well blended. Remove from heat and reserve for serving.
In a small bowl mix together the flour, paprika,
cayenne pepper and salt. Place chicken wings in a large
nonporous glass dish or bowl and sprinkle flour mixture over
them until they are evenly coated. Cover dish or bowl and
refrigerate for 60 to 90 minutes.
Fry coated wings in hot oil for 10 to 15 minutes,
or until parts of wings begin to turn brown.
Remove from heat, place wings in serving bowl,
add hot sauce mixture and stir together. Serve.

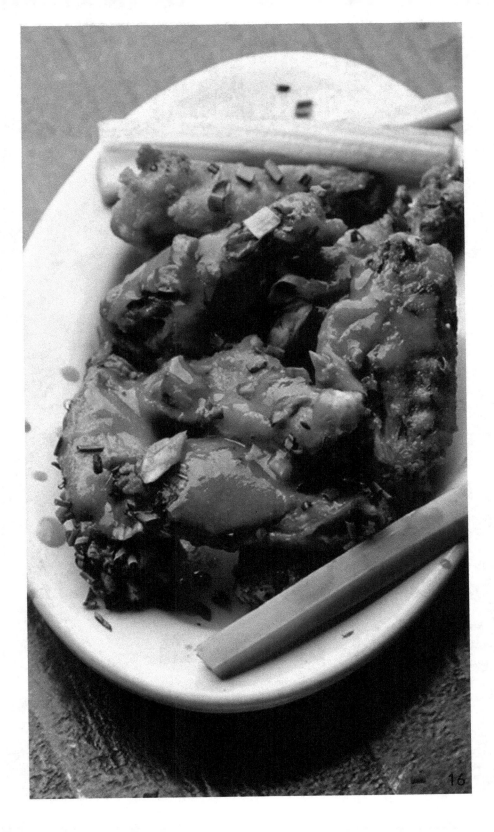

Special Honey BBQ Sauce

2 cloves garlic, minced | 1 tablespoon minced shallot

1/2 cup honey | 2 cups barbecue sauce, your choice

3 tablespoons chopped fresh cilantro

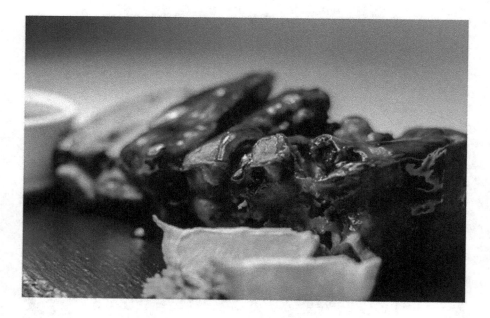

Directions:

In a medium, nonporous bowl,
combine the garlic, shallot, honey, barbecue sauce and cilantro.
Mix well and pour onto meat or poultry.
Discard any leftover sauce.

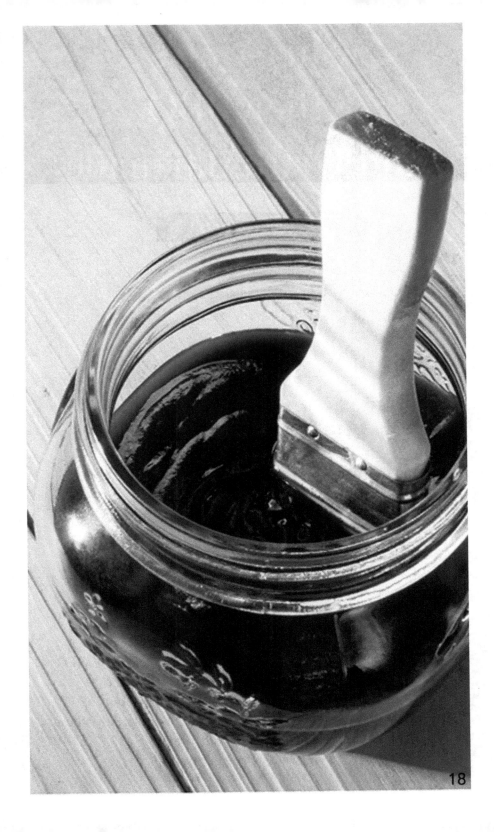

Christian's Killer BBQ and Grill Marinade

Ingredients:

1/3 cup apple cider vinegar

1/4 cup Worcestershire sauce

1/4 cup soy sauce

1/4 cup honey

1/4 cup molasses

1/4 cup whiskey

1/3 cup seasoning salt

1/3 cup salt-free seasoning blend

1/4 cup garlic powder

1 tablespoon ginger

2 tablespoons browning sauce

2 tablespoons prepared mustard

1 tablespoon hickory-flavored liquid smoke

Directions:

Place oil, vinegar, Worcestershire sauce, soy sauce, honey,
molasses, whiskey, seasoning salt, salt-free seasoning blend,
garlic powder, ginger, browning sauce, mustard,
and liquid smoke in a resealable container or bottle,
and shake well. Store marinade in refrigerator until ready to use.
Bring marinade to room temperature and
shake well before each use.

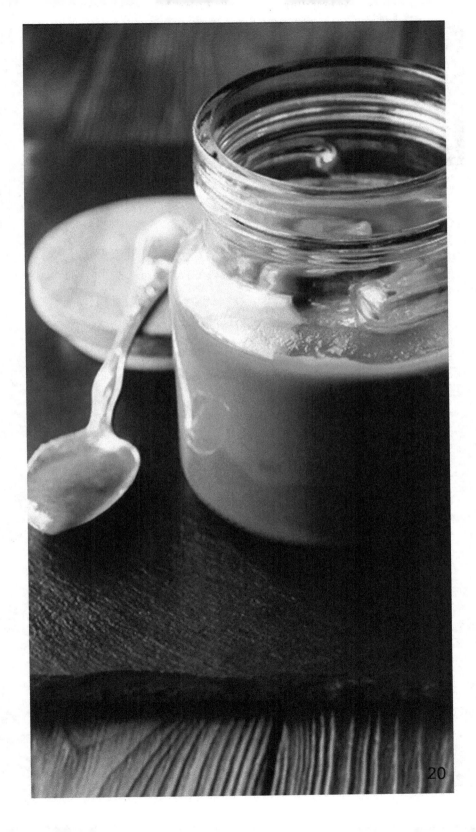

Grilled Spice Rubbed Chicken Breasts

Ingredients:

1 cup Hellmann's® or Best Foods® Real Mayonnaise

2 tablespoons cider vinegar

2 tablespoons horseradish

1/8 teaspoon cayenne chili powder

4 (6 ounce) boneless, skinless chicken breasts

2 tablespoons canola oil

2 tablespoons Bobby Flay's Sixteen Spice Rub for Poultry or your favorite spice rub or grill seasoning

Directions:

Combine Hellmann's® or Best Foods® Real Mayonnaise, vinegar, horseradish and chili powder in small bowl.
Season, if desired, with salt and pepper; reserve 1/2 cup sauce and set aside.
Brush chicken on both sides with oil and season, if desired, with salt and pepper.
Evenly sprinkle top of chicken with spice rub.
Grill chicken, rub-side down, until golden brown and crust has formed, about 4 minutes.
Brush chicken with mayonnaise mixture, turn over and cook an additional 4 minutes or until chicken is thoroughly cooked. Remove to serving platter, t hen cover loosely with aluminum foil and let sit 5 minutes before serving.
Slice each breast and serve with reserved 1/2 cup sauce on the side.

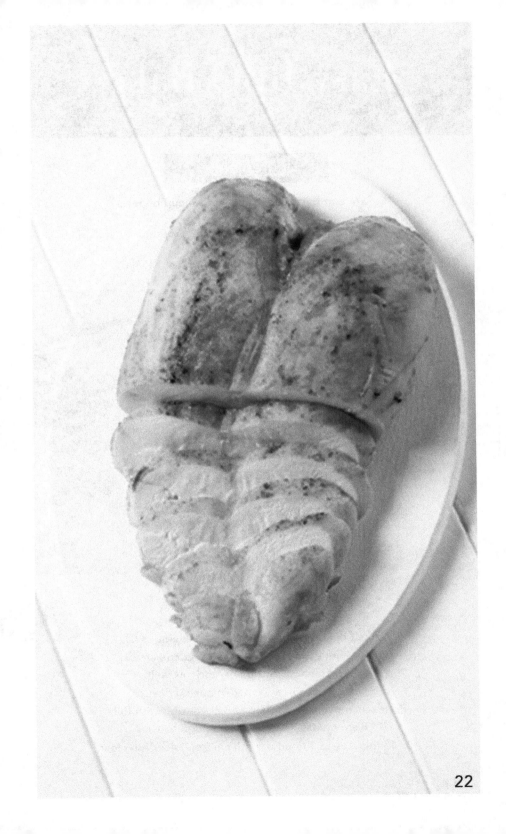

Easy BBQ Bake

3/4 cup barbecue sauce | 3/4 cup honey

1/2 cup ketchup | 1 onion, chopped

4 skinless, boneless chicken breast halves

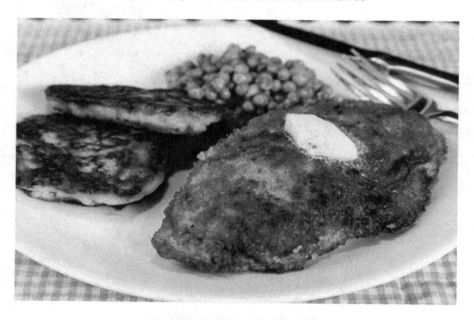

Preheat oven to 400 degrees F (200 degrees C).
In a medium bowl, combine the barbecue sauce,
honey, ketchup and onion and mix well.
Place chicken in a 9x13 inch baking dish.
Pour sauce over the chicken and cover dish with foil.
Bake at 400 degrees F (200 degrees C)
for 45 minutes to 1 hour, or until chicken juices run clear.

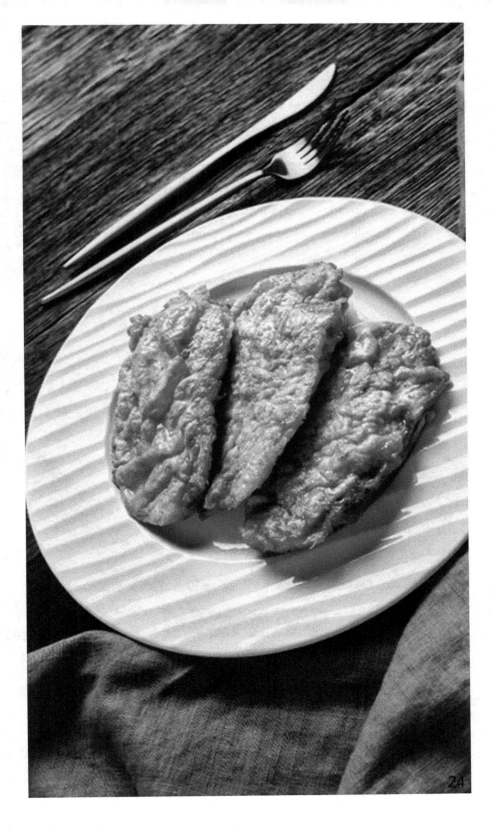

Kowloon's Chinese Chicken Wings

Ingredients:

3 pounds chicken wings | 3 tablespoons salt

2 tablespoons white sugar | 6 tablespoons water

6 tablespoons soy sauce | 1 tablespoon gin

1/4 teaspoon ground ginger | 1 quart vegetable oil for frying

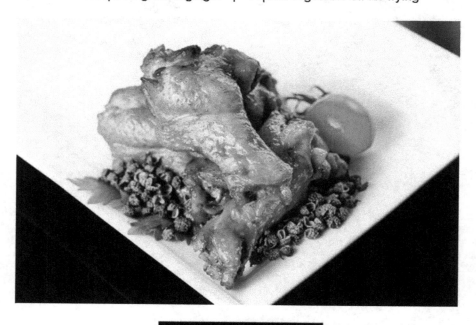

Directions:

FOR MARINADE:
Combine the salt, sugar, water, soy sauce, gin and ginger.
Put mixture in a zipper style plastic bag, add chicken
and marinate for 24 hours or as long as possible, turning bag frequently.
In a large skillet over medium high heat fry marinated chicken wings
in hot oil until golden brown,
about 8 minutes each side. Ready to serve!

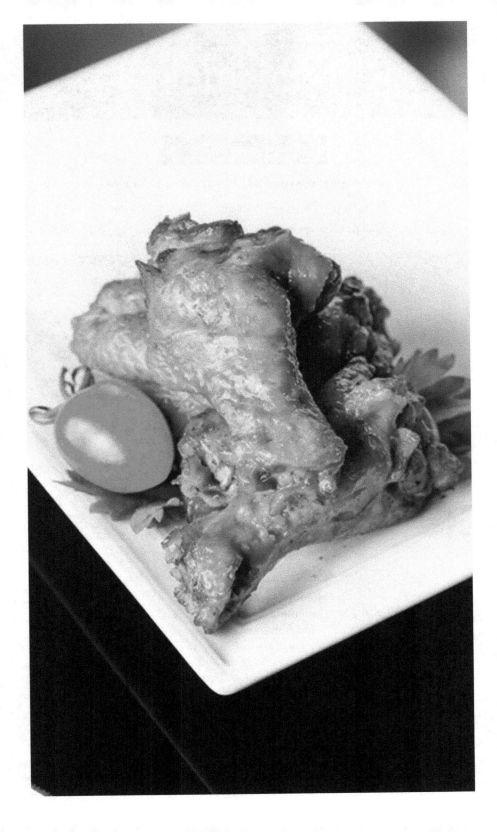

BBQ Chicken

3 tablespoons vegetable oil | 1 1/2 cups cider vinegar

1 tablespoon salt | 1/4 teaspoon ground black pepper

2 teaspoons poultry seasoning | 2 pounds cut up chicken pieces

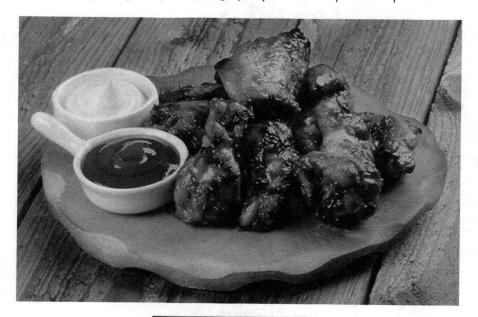

Directions:

Heat grill to medium heat.
In a small skillet combine the oil, vinegar, salt and pepper
and put over low heat.
Add the poultry seasoning while stirring constantly;
when sauce mixes well and starts to bubble, it is done.
Place chicken on hot grill and brush with sauce.
Grill for 45 to 60 minutes, turning every 5 to 10 minutes,
and brush chicken with sauce after each turning.
Grill until chicken is done and juices run clear.
(Note: Be sure to keep an eye on the chicken as it cooks,
as it tends to have flair ups due to the oil and chicken drippings!)

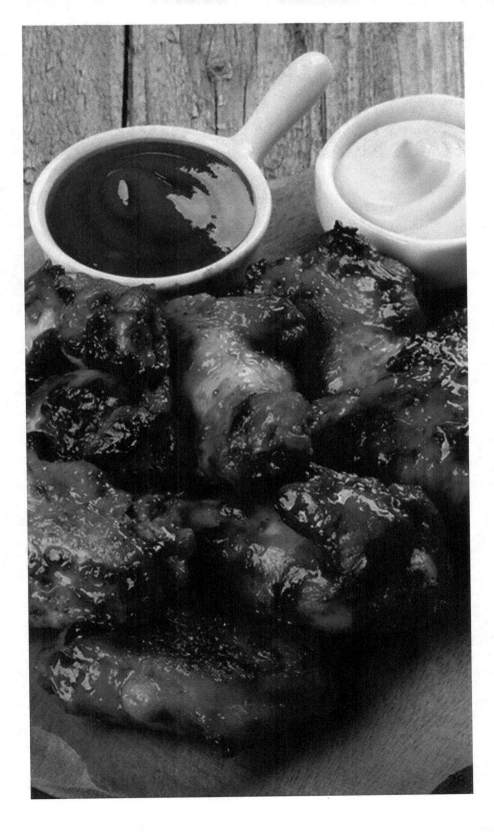

Tex-Mex Chicken Salad

Ingredients:

2 pounds skinless, boneless chicken breasts

½ cup chopped jalapeno pepper | 1 green onion, sliced

2 tablespoons butter

2 (8 ounce) cartons Lucerne Whipped Cream Cheese Spread

1 (14.5 ounce) can diced tomatoes | 1/2 cup salsa

1/2 teaspoon salt Shredded lettuce | 1 cup shredded Monterey Jack cheese

1 (4 ounce) can sliced ripe olives, drained | 3 cups crushed tortilla chips

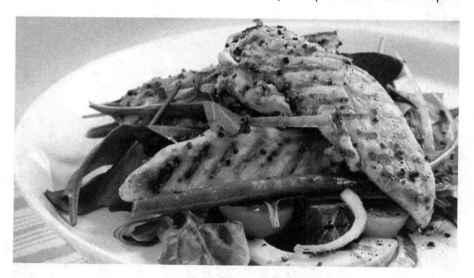

Directions:

In a large skillet, saute the chicken,
jalapenos and onion in butter until chicken is no longer pink.
Add the cream cheese, tomatoes, salsa and salt; stir until blended.
Serve over lettuce; sprinkle with cheese, olives and tortilla chips.

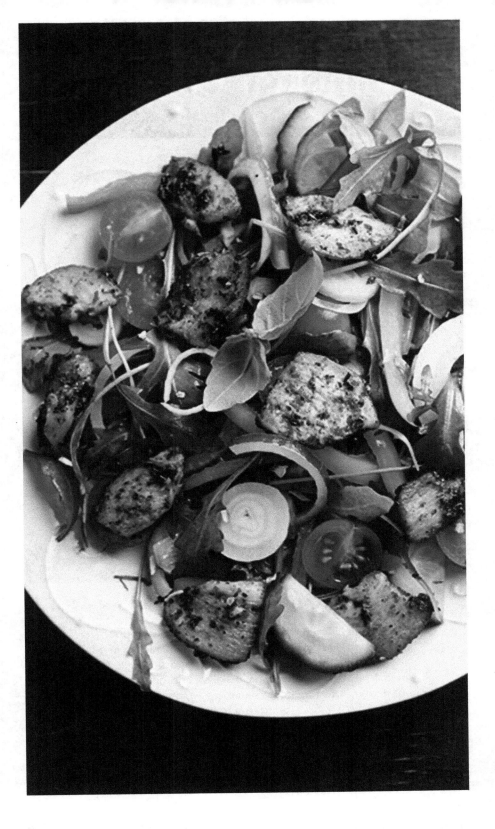

Chicken Confetti

1 (3 pound) broiler-fryer chicken, cut up 1 teaspoon salt, divided

1/4 teaspoon pepper | 2 tablespoons cooking oil

1 medium onion, chopped | 1 garlic clove, minced

2 (14.5 ounce) cans diced tomatoes, undrained

1 (8 ounce) can tomato sauce | 1 (6 ounce) can tomato paste

1 1/2 teaspoons dried basil

1 (7 ounce) package spaghetti, cooked and drained

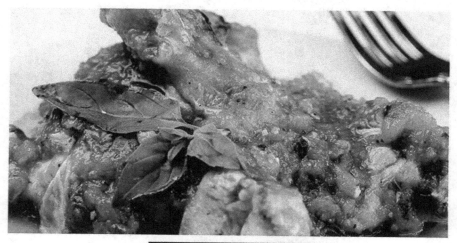

Directions:

Sprinkle chicken with 1/2 teaspoon salt and pepper.
In a large skillet over medium heat, brown chicken in oil.
Remove chicken and set aside.
Reserve 1 tablespoon drippings in skillet; add onion and garlic.
Saute until tender. Add tomatoes, sauce, paste, basil and remaining salt;
bring to a boil.
Return chicken to skillet. Reduce heat;
cover and simmer for 60-70 minutes or until meat is tender
Serve over spaghetti.

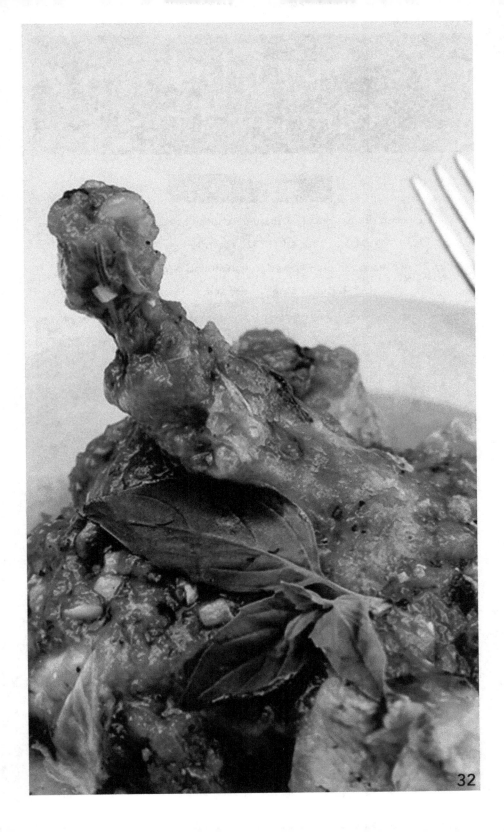

32

Spicy Hot Chicken Legs

Ingredients:

12 chicken drumsticks | 1 (5 ounce) bottle hot red pepper sauce

1/4 cup butter, cubed | 1/2 teaspoon garlic powder

1/2 teaspoon onion powder | salt and pepper to taste

1 1/2 cups blue cheese salad dressing

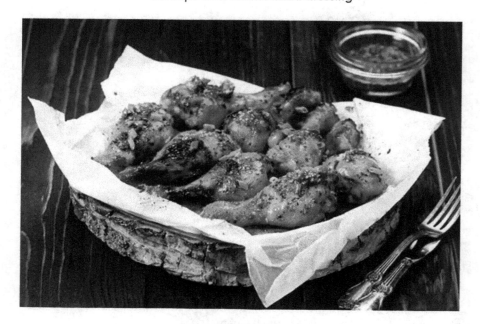

Directions:

Place the drumsticks in a slow cooker, and sprinkle evenly
with pieces of butter. Pour the hot sauce over the chicken,
then season with garlic powder, onion powder, salt and pepper.
Cover, and cook on High for 3 hours, or until tender.
Serve chicken legs with blue cheese dressing on the side.

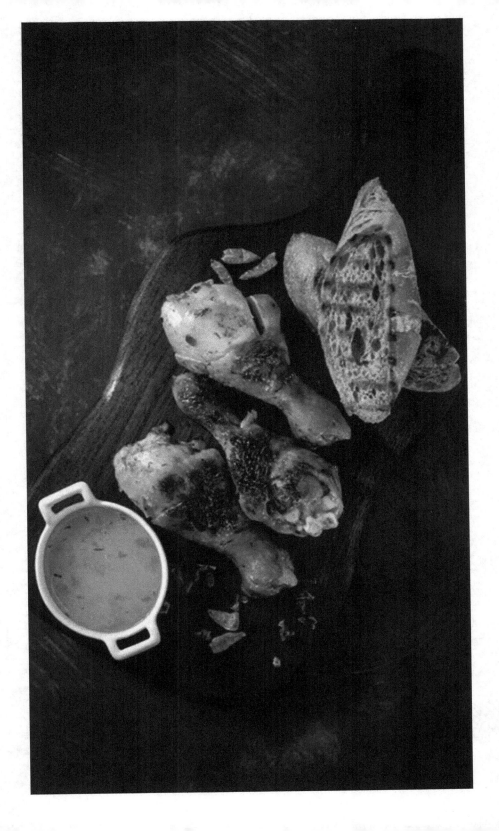

Honey Baked Chicken

Ingredients:

1 (3 pound) whole chicken, cut into pieces | 1/2 cup butter, melted

1/2 cup honey | 1/4 cup prepared mustard

1 teaspoon salt | 1 teaspoon curry powder

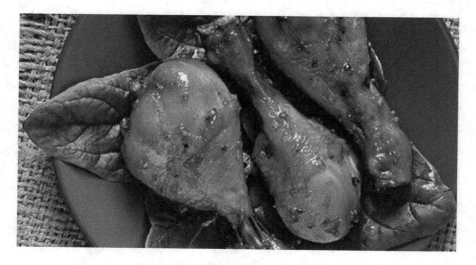

Directions:

Preheat oven to 350 degrees F (175 degrees C).

Place chicken pieces in a shallow baking pan, skin side up.

Combine the melted butter or margarine, honey, mustard, salt
and curry powder and pour the mixture over the chicken.

Bake in the preheated oven for 1 1/4 hours (75 minutes),
basting every 15 minutes with pan drippings, until
the chicken is nicely browned and tender and the juices run clear.

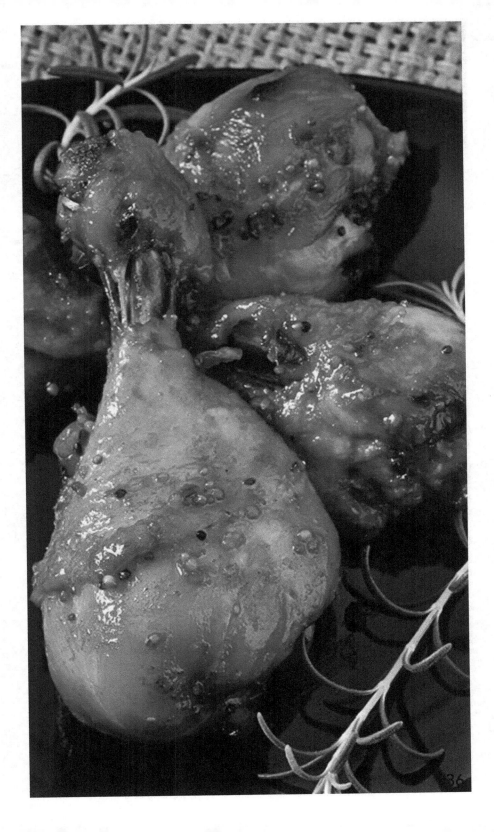

Chicken Salad Oriental

1 1/2 cups cubed cooked chicken | 1 1/2 cups cooked rice

1 (10 ounce) package frozen green beans, thawed | 1 cup fresh bean sprouts

1 medium green pepper, chopped | 1 small onion, chopped

2 tablespoons minced fresh parsley

DRESSING:

1/3 cup sour cream | 2 tablespoons water

2 tablespoons soy sauce | 1/2 teaspoon garlic powder

1/2 teaspoon salt | 1/4 teaspoon ground ginger

1/8 teaspoon pepper

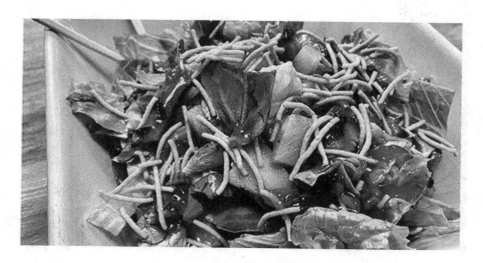

Directions:

In a large bowl, combine the first seven ingredients.
Whisk dressing ingredients together in a small bowl.
Pour over salad; toss to coat. Refrigerate 8 hour or overnight.

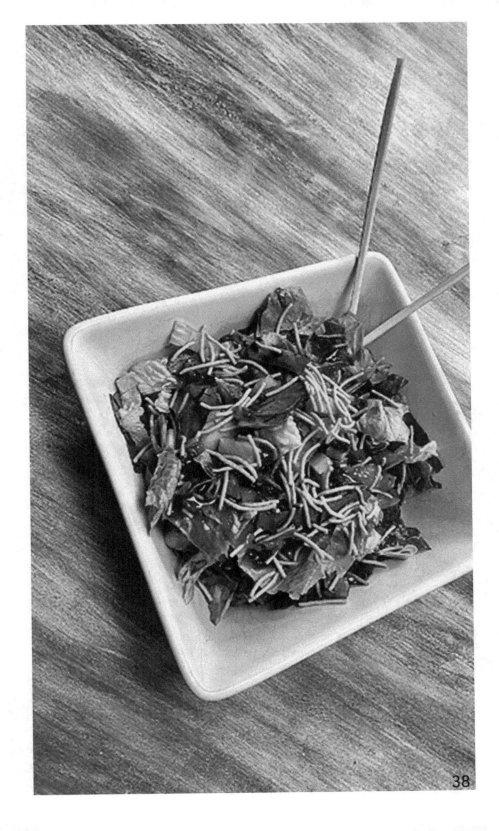

Lime-Garlic Chicken and Spinach Salad

Ingredients:

4 skinless, boneless chicken breast halves - cut into thin strips

L   1/2 onion, chopped | 2 tablespoons minced garlic

1 teaspoon fresh ground black pepper | 1 pinch salt

1 teaspoon flour | 1/4 cup fresh lime juice, or to taste

4 1/2 cups baby spinach leaves

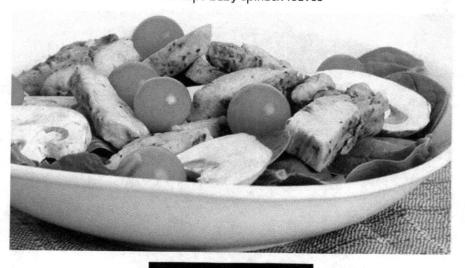

Directions:

Place chicken, onions, garlic, salt, pepper,
and flour in a resealable bag.
Stir in the lime juice.
Allow to sit for a few minutes to marinate.
Spray a non-stick frying pan with olive oil cooking spray
and place over medium heat.
Pour in the entire contents of the bag and cook
until the onion has softened (there is no need to brown).
Add additional lime juice to taste. Serve over spinach.

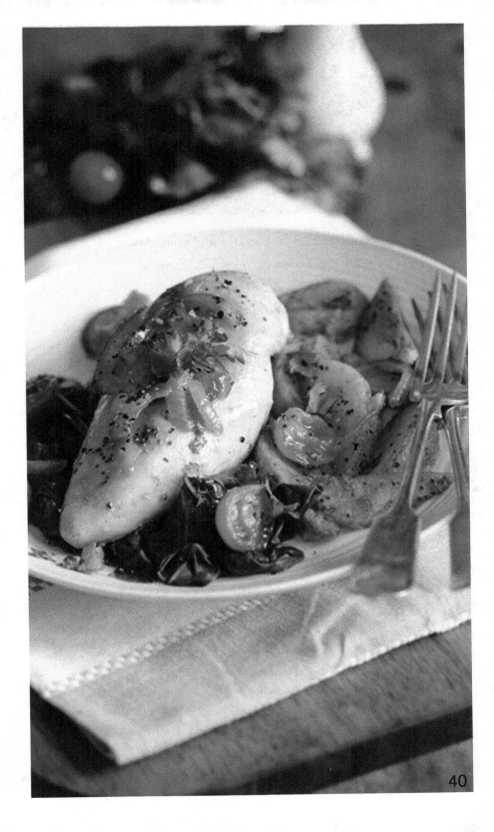

Chicken Pasta Salad

1/2 pound uncooked pasta of your choice

1 cup frozen corn kernels, thawed

1 cup sliced mushrooms

1/2 cup diced celery

1/4 cup minced onion

1/2 cup sliced green olives

1/2 cup diced green bell pepper

1 cup shredded Cheddar cheese

3/4 cup Italian-style salad dressing

1/2 cup mayonnaise

2 (10 ounce) cans chunk chicken, drained

salt and pepper to taste

Directions:

Bring a large pot of lightly salted water to a boil.
Add pasta and cook for 8 to 10 minutes or until al dente;
drain and pour pasta into a large dish.
Stir in the corn, mushrooms, celery, onions, olives,
bell pepper and cheese.
In a separate bowl, whisk together the salad dressing
and mayonnaise, then pour this mixture over the salad
and toss again, to coat.
Add flaked chicken and toss gently a final time.

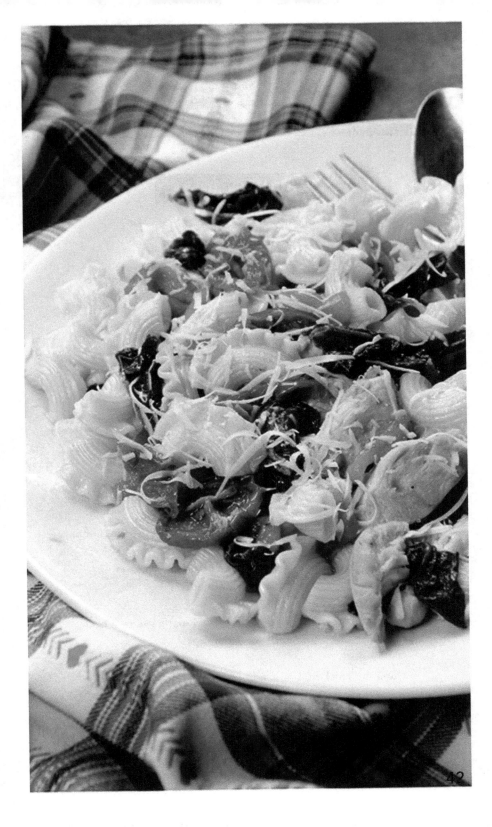

Orange Teriyaki Chicken

Ingredients:

4 bone-in chicken breast halves, with skin

1/3 cup teriyaki sauce

1/3 (12 fluid ounce) can frozen orange juice concentrate, thawed

Directions:

Rinse chicken breasts. Pat dry with paper towels.
Place in a plastic bag set into a shallow dish.

TO MAKE MARINADE:
Combine teriyaki sauce and orange juice concentrate.

Pour marinade over the chicken and close the plastic bag.

Marinate in the refrigerator for 6 to 24 hours, turning occasionally.

Remove from refrigerator and drain the chicken,
reserving the marinade.

In a small saucepan, bring the reserved marinade to a boil
and cook for 2 minutes.

Grill the chicken, bone side up, on an uncovered grill
directly over medium coals for 20 minutes.

Turn the chicken and grill for 20 to 30 minutes more or until tender,
brushing often with the reserved marinade. Serve.

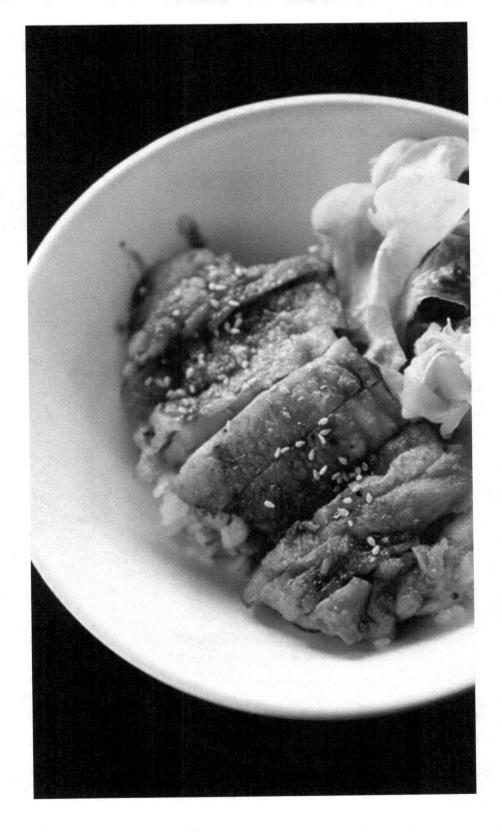

BBQ Meatballs

1 (16 ounce) package frozen meatballs

1 (18 ounce) bottle barbecue sauce | 1/4 cup ketchup

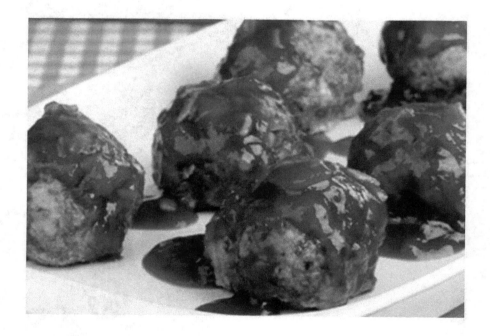

Directions:

Place prepared meatballs, barbeque sauce,
and ketchup in a slow cooker.

Let it cook on a low heat for 4 hours, stirring occasionally.

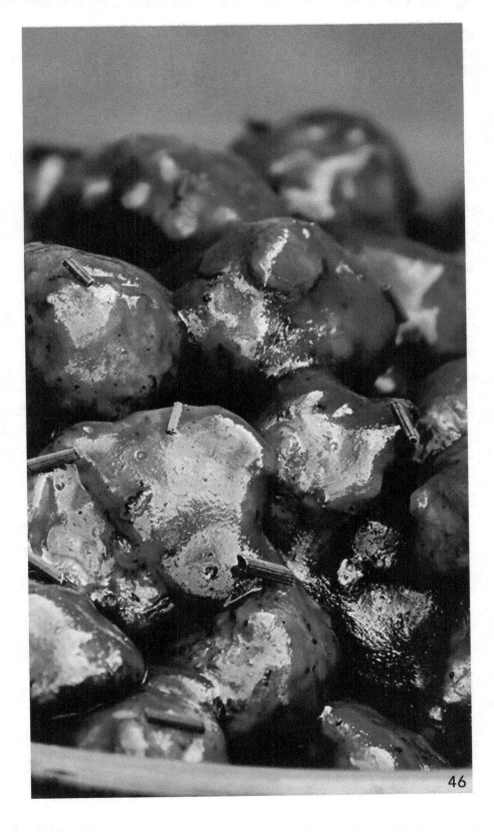

Marinade for Chicken

1 1/2 cups vegetable oil | 3/4 cup soy sauce

1/2 cup Worcestershire sauce | 1/2 cup red wine vinegar

1/3 cup lemon juice | 2 tablespoons dry mustard

1 teaspoon salt | 1 tablespoon black pepper

1 1/2 teaspoons finely minced fresh parsley

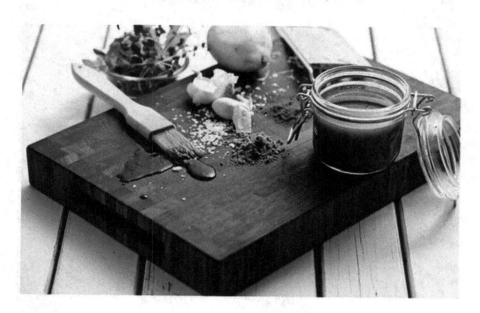

Directions:

In a medium bowl, mix together oil, soy sauce,
Worcestershire sauce, wine vinegar, and lemon juice.
Stir in mustard powder, salt, pepper, and parsley.
Use to marinate chicken before cooking as desired.
The longer you marinate, the more flavor it will have.

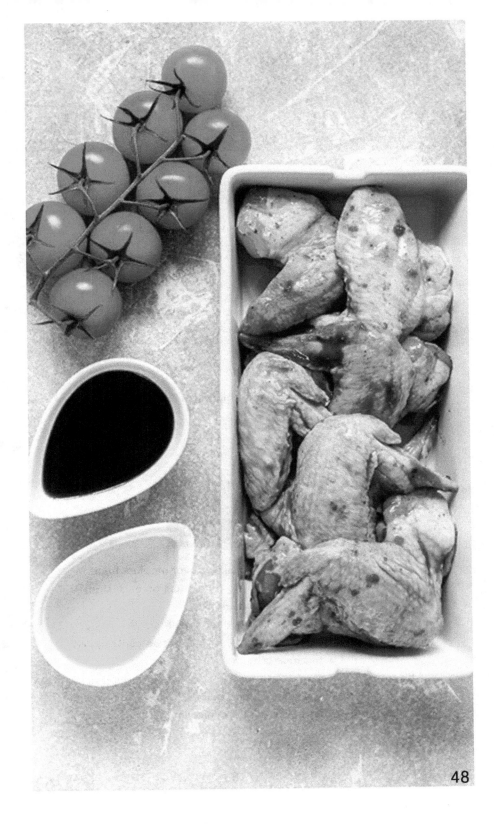

Fresh Chicken Salad with Baby Greens

2 tablespoons extra virgin olive oil, divided

2 skinless, boneless chicken breast halves

1/4 cup pesto sauce

3 cups mixed baby greens

1 medium red bell pepper, sliced

1 small cucumber, sliced

1/4 red onion, thinly sliced

1 tablespoon balsamic vinegar

1 tablespoon honey

salt and pepper to taste

Directions:

Heat 1 tablespoon olive oil in a skillet over medium heat.
Cook chicken breast in the skillet 10 minutes on each side,
or until juices run clear.
Remove chicken from skillet and shred.
Return to skillet, mix in pesto sauce, and continue cooking just
until sauce is heated through.
Place greens in a bowl, and top with chicken, bell pepper,
cucumber, and onion.
Drizzle with remaining olive oil, balsamic vinegar, and honey.
Season with salt and pepper.
Toss, and serve

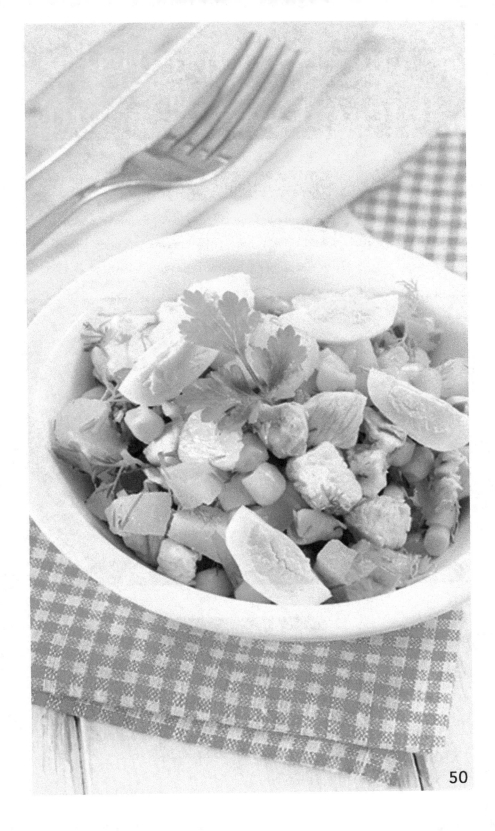

Angela's Oriental Chicken Noodle Soup

3 cups water | 1 (3 ounce) package chicken flavored ramen noodles

2 cups chopped cooked chicken breast | 2 leaves bok choy, sliced

1 carrot, sliced | 1 teaspoon sesame oil

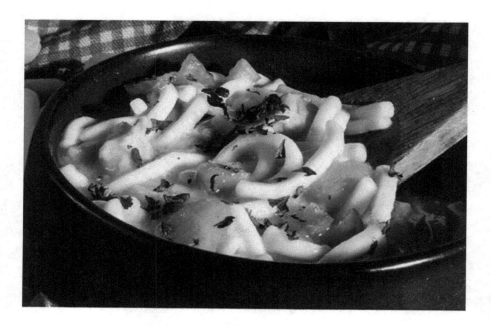

Directions:

In a large saucepan, bring water to a boil.
Break up block of noodles and stir into pot,
reserving seasoning packet.
Stir in chicken, bok choy and carrot.
Bring to a boil again, then reduce heat and simmer 3 minutes.
Stir in contents of seasoning packet and sesame oil.

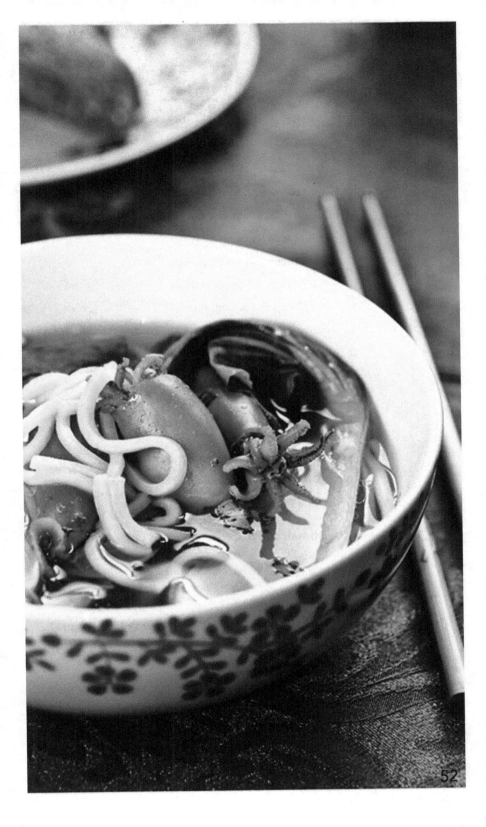

Chicken Pepper Steak

Ingredients:

1 tablespoon vegetable oil

4 boneless, skinless chicken breasts

1 teaspoon seasoning salt

1/2 teaspoon onion powder

2 teaspoons minced garlic

1/2 cup soy sauce, divided

1 large onion, cut into long slices

2 tablespoons cornstarch

2 1/2 cups water

1 green bell pepper, sliced

4 roma (plum) tomatoes, seeded and chopped

Directions:

Heat oil in a large skillet over medium heat.

Season chicken with salt and onion powder, and place in skillet.

Cook for about 5 to 7 minutes, then add the garlic,
4 tablespoons soy sauce, and half of the sliced onion.

Cook until chicken is no longer pink, and the juices run clear.

Dissolve cornstarch in water in a small bowl,and blend into
the chicken mixture.

Stir in 4 tablespoons soy sauce, bell pepper,
tomatoes, and remaining onion.

Simmer until gravy has reached desired consistency

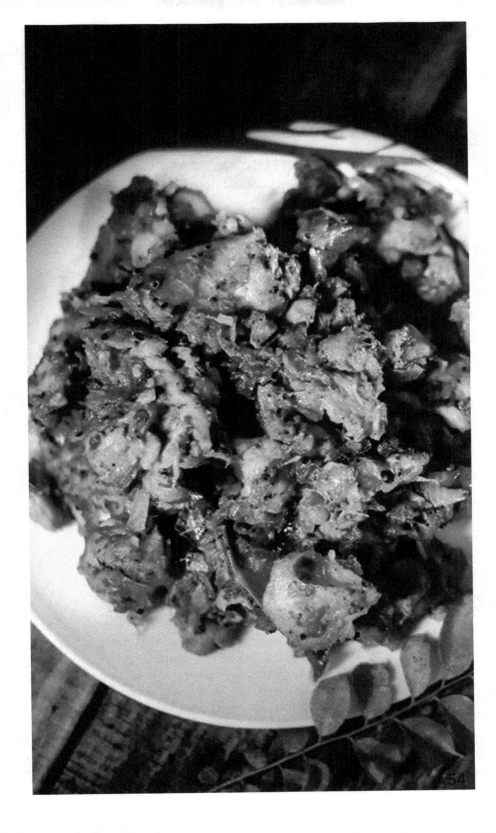

Pumpkin Mousse Cheesecake

Ingredients:

1 cup graham cracker crumbs

3 tablespoons sugar

1/4 cup butter or margarine, melted

3 (8 ounce) packages cream cheese, softened

1 cup sugar 1 cup canned pumpkin

3 tablespoons all-purpose flour

1 teaspoon ground cinnamon

1/4 teaspoon ground nutmeg

4 eggs

Directions:

Combine crumbs, sugar and butter.
Press into a greased 9-in. springform pan.
Bake at 325 degrees F for 8 minutes.
Cool on a wire rack.

Meanwhile, in a mixing bowl, beat cream cheese
and sugar until smooth.
Add pumpkin, flour, cinnamon and nutmeg.
Add eggs; beat on low speed just until combined.
Pour into crust.
Bake for 50 minutes or until center is almost set.
Cool on a wire rack for 10 minutes.
Carefully run a knife around edge of pan to loosen;
cool 1 hour longer. Refrigerate overnight.
In a saucepan over low heat, melt chips and shortening;
stir until smooth.
Drizzle over cheesecake. Refrigerate until firm,
about 30 minutes.

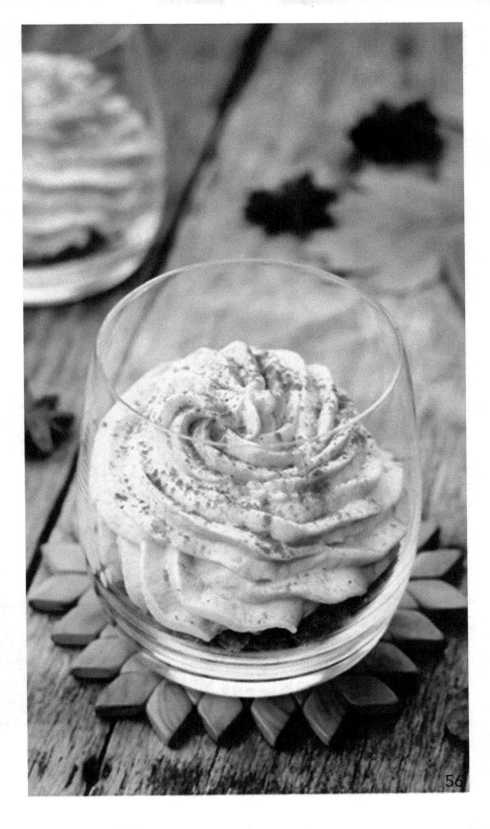

Sunflower Cheese Ball

Ingredients:

1 (8 ounce) package cream cheese, softened | 1 teaspoon Dijon mustard

1/2 teaspoon garlic powder | 2 cups shredded Cheddar cheese

1/2 cup chopped ripe olives | 2 tablespoons minced fresh parsley

1/2 cup salted sunflower kernels assorted crackers

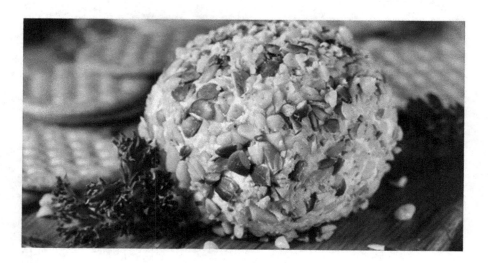

In

White Bean Fennel Soup

Shape into a ball; roll in sunflower kernels.

Store in the refrige

Ingredients:

1 large onion, chopped

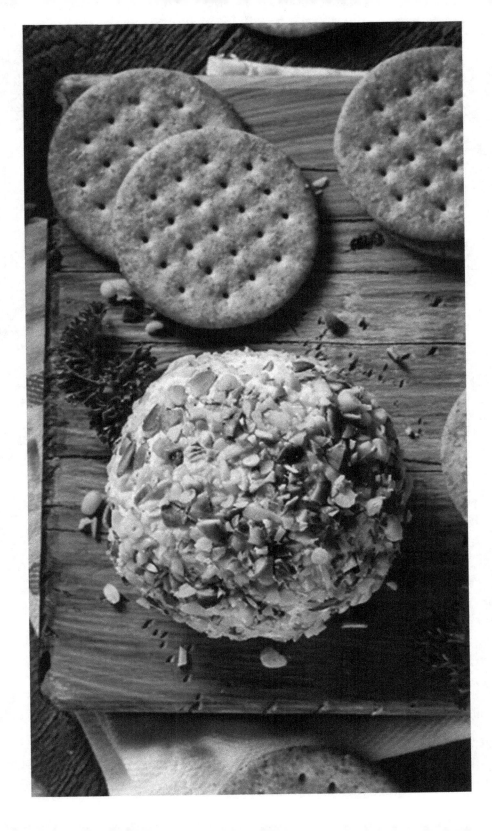

Smoked Beef Brisket

Ingredients:

2 1/2 pounds beef brisket | 1 tablespoon liquid smoke flavoring

1 teaspoon salt | 1/2 teaspoon pepper

1/2 cup chopped onion | 1/2 cup ketchup

2 teaspoons Dijon mustard | 1/2 teaspoon celery seed

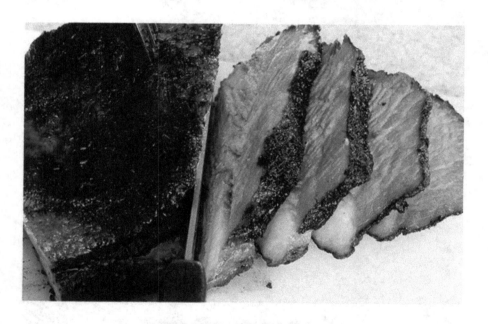

Directions:

Cut the brisket in half; rub with Liquid Smoke, salt and pepper.
Place in a 3-qt. slow cooker. Top with onion.
Combine the ketchup, mustard and celery seed; spread over meat.
Cover and cook on low for 8-9 hours. Remove brisket and keep warm.
Transfer cooking juices to a blender; cover and process until smooth.
Serve with brisket.

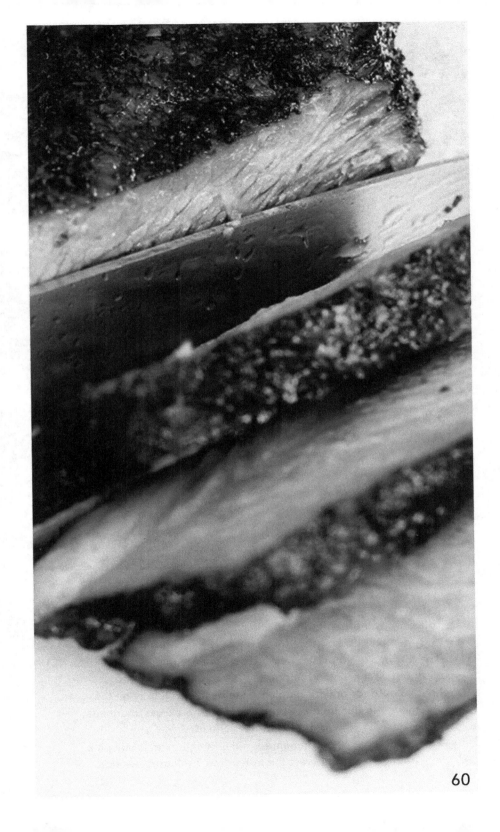

Kalbi Korean BBQ Short Ribs)

3/4 cup soy sauce | 3/4 cup brown sugar

3/4 cup water | 1 garlic clove, minced

2 green onions, chopped | 1 tablespoon Asian (toasted)

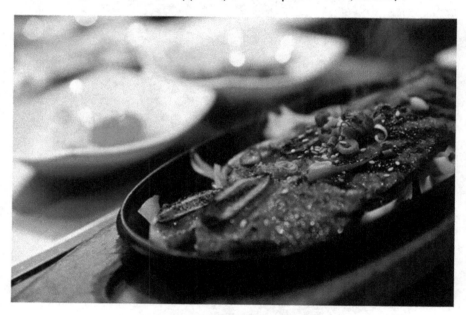

Directions:

In a bowl, stir together the soy sauce, brown sugar, water, garlic,
green onions, and sesame oil until the sugar has dissolved.
Place the ribs in a large plastic zipper bag. Pour the marinade over the ribs,
squeeze out all the air, and refrigerate the bag for 3 hours to overnight.
Preheat an outdoor grill for medium-high heat, and lightly oil the grate.
Remove the ribs from the bag, shake off the excess marinade,
and discard the marinade.
Grill the ribs on the preheated grill until the meat is still pink
but not bloody nearest the bone, 5 to 7 minutes per side.

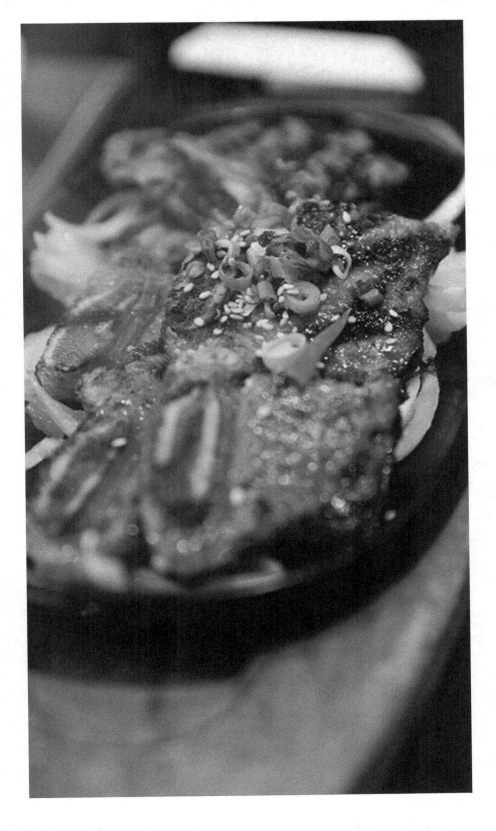

Spaghetti Sauce with Ground Beef

Ingredients:

1 pound ground beef | 1 onion, chopped

4 cloves garlic, minced | 1 small green bell pepper, diced

1 (28 ounce) can diced tomatoes | 1 (16 ounce) can tomato sauce

1 (6 ounce) can tomato paste | 2 teaspoons dried oregano

2 teaspoons dried basil | 1 teaspoon salt

1/2 teaspoon black pepper

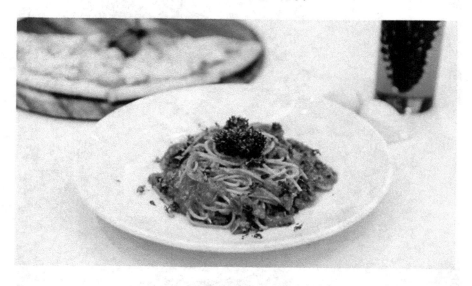

Directions:

Combine ground beef, onion, garlic, and green pepper in a large saucepan.
Cook and stir until meat is brown and vegetables are tender. Drain grease.
Stir diced tomatoes, tomato sauce, and tomato paste into the pan.
Season with oregano, basil, salt, and pepper.
Simmer spaghetti sauce for 1 hour, stirring occasionally.

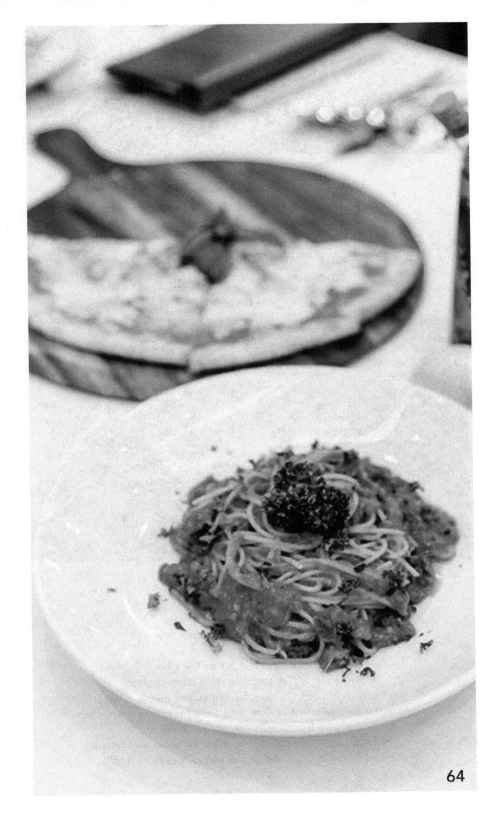

Slow Cooker
Baked Beans

Ingredients:

24 ounces dry white beans | 1 pound ham hocks

1 onion, chopped | 1/2 cup packed brown sugar

1/2 cup maple syrup | 1 teaspoon salt

1 cup water | 1/2 cup ketchup

2 tablespoons prepared mustard

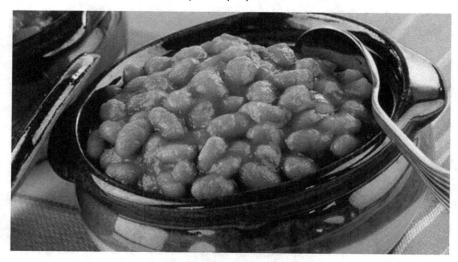

Directions:

In a large pot over high heat,
combine the beans with water to cover and
bring to a boil for 10 minutes.
Remove from heat but let sit for 1 hour.
Drain beans and place them in a slow cooker.
Add the ham hocks, onion, brown sugar, maple syrup,
salt and water. Mix well, cover and cook on high setting for
4 to 5 hours, stirring occasionally.
During the final hour of cooking, add the ketchup and mustard,
remove the ham from the hocks and discard the hocks.
Mix well and serve.

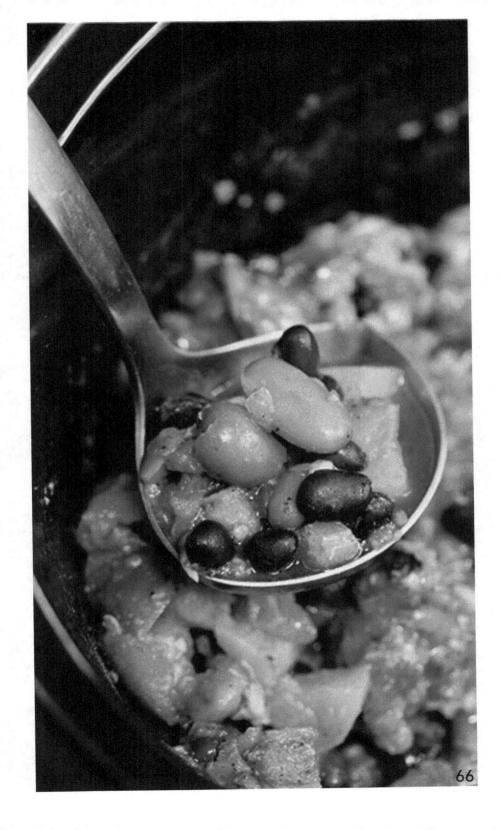

White Bean Fennel Soup

Ingredients:

1 large onion, chopped

1 small fennel bulb, thinly sliced

1 tablespoon olive oil

5 cups reduced sodium chicken broth or
vegetable broth

1 (15 ounce) can white kidney or

cannelini beans, rinsed and drained

1 (14.5 ounce) can diced tomatoes, undrained

1 teaspoon dried thyme

1/4 teaspoon pepper

1 bay leaf

3 cups shredded fresh spinach

Directions:

In a large saucepan, saute onion and
fennel in oil until tender.

Add the broth, beans, tomatoes,
thyme, pepper and bay leaf; bring to a boil.

Reduce heat; cover and simmer for 30 minutes or
until fennel is tender.

Discard bay leaf. Add spinach;
cook 3-4 minutes longer or until spinach is wilted.

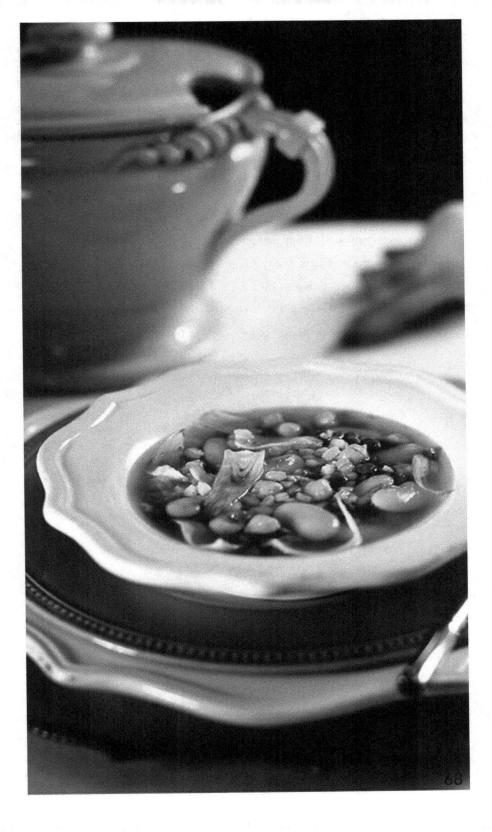

Feta and Slow-Roasted Tomato Salad with French

Ingredients:

12 cherry tomatoes salt and black pepper to taste

1/4 cup olive oil 1 bay leaf, crumbled | 1/4 cup pine nuts

2/3 pound thin green beans, trimmed | 1 (5 ounce) package arugula leaves

6 fresh basil leaves, torn into pieces | 1 tablespoon red wine vinegar

2 tablespoons whole-grain mustard | 2 cloves garlic, minced

1/2 teaspoon honey | 1/4 cup olive oil

6 ounces crumbled feta cheese

Directions:

Preheat an oven to 225 degrees F (110 degrees C).
Slice the cherry tomatoes in half, and arrange them, cut sides up,
on a baking sheet. Sprinkle them with salt, pepper, and
the bay leaf;drizzle with 1/4 cup olive oil.
Bake the tomatoes until they are shriveled and dry on the
outside, but a little moist inside, about 2 hours.
Toast the pine nuts in a small pan over medium-low heat,
gently shaking the pan as they toast,
until beginning brown and fragrant, 2 to 3 minutes; set aside.
Bring a saucepan of water to a boil;
cook the green beans in the boiling water until
bright green but still crisp, about 3 minutes.
Drain and rinse immediately with cold water.
Combine the roasted tomatoes, toasted pine nuts,
green beans, arugula, and basil in a salad bowl.
Whisk together the red wine vinegar, mustard, garlic, honey,
and 1/4 cup olive oil in a bowl,
and pour the dressing over the salad.
Stir in the crumbled feta cheese just before serving.

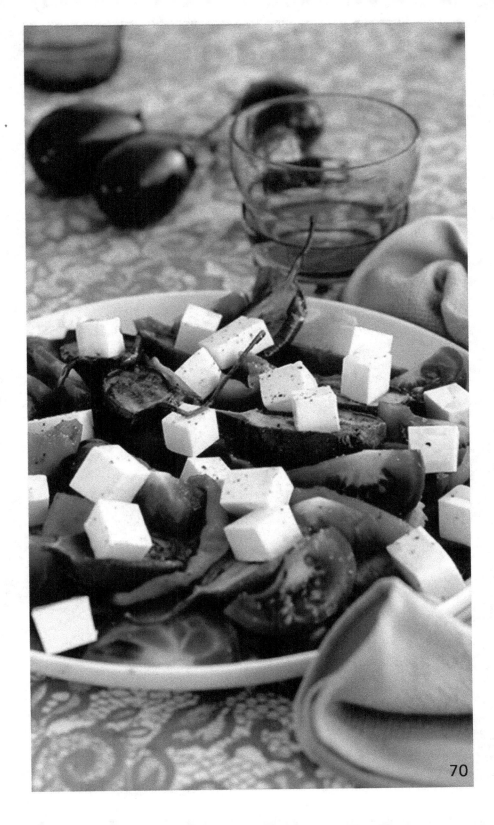

Cucumber and Tomato Salad

1 tomato, chopped | 1 cucumber, seeded and chopped
1/4 cup thinly sliced red onion | 1/4 cup canned kidney beans, drained
1/4 cup diced firm tofu | 2 tablespoons chopped fresh basil
1/4 cup balsamic vinaigrette salad dressing | salt and pepper to taste

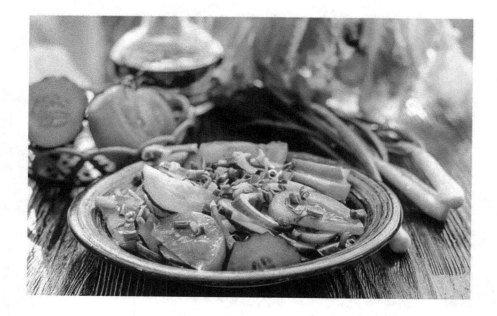

Directions:

In a large bowl, combine the tomato, cucumber, red onion,
kidney beans, tofu, and basil.
Just before serving, toss with balsamic vinaigrette salad dressing,
and season with salt and pepper.

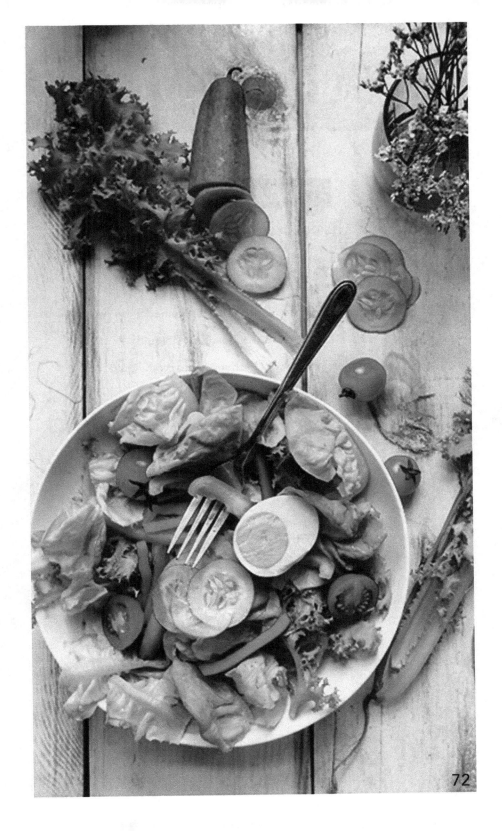

Beans and Greens

4 (14.5 ounce) cans vegetable broth

1 (10 ounce) package frozen chopped spinach

1 (15 ounce) can dark red kidney beans, drained and rinsed

1 (15 ounce) can light red kidney beans, drained and rinsed

1 (15 ounce) can black beans, with liquid

1 (15 ounce) can great Northern beans, with liquid

1 (15 ounce) can pinto beans, with liquid

1/4 cup vegetable oil

1 tablespoon garlic powder salt to taste

black pepper to taste

Directions:

Place broth and spinach in a pot over medium heat,
and cook 5 minutes, or until spinach is thawed.

Mix in dark and light kidney beans, black beans and liquid,
great northern beans and liquid, pinto beans and liquid, and oil.

Season with garlic powder, salt, and pepper.

Cook 30 minutes, stirring occasionally.

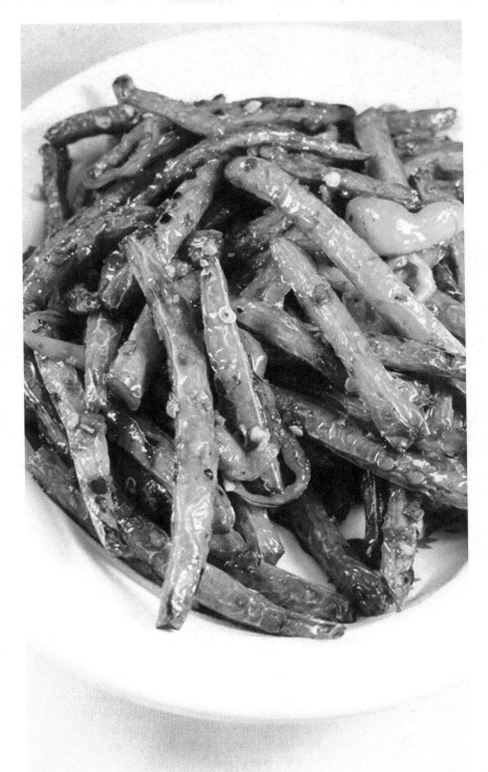

Scottie's Chicken Tortilla Soup

Ingredients:

1 (49.5 fluid ounce) can chicken broth

1 (14 ounce) can whole kernel corn, drained

1 (14 ounce) can black beans, drained

1 cube beef bouillon | 3/4 cup chopped broccoli

1 (28 ounce) can stewed tomatoes (crushed) | 2 tablespoons olive oil

8 corn tortillas, cut into 1-inch strips | 2 tablespoons olive oil

2 boneless skinless chicken breasts, cut into 1/2 inch cubes

2 tablespoons lime juice 1 tablespoon tequila

1 tablespoon onion powder | 1 tablespoon garlic salt

1 tablespoon cayenne pepper | 2 tablespoons Cajun seasoning

1 cup shredded white Cheddar cheese

Directions:

Combine the chicken broth, corn, black beans, beef bouillon,
broccoli, and tomatoes in a large pot over medium heat.
While the broth mixture simmers, heat 2 tablespoons olive oil
in a skillet. Fry the tortilla strips in the hot oil until crisp.
Remove from skillet and drain on paper towels.
Pour 2 tablespoons olive oil into the skillet.
Once the oil is hot, add the chicken; cook and stir until
cooked through, about 5 minutes.
Stir in the lime juice, tequila, onion powder, garlic salt,
cayenne pepper, and Cajun seasoning; cook another 2 minutes.
Transfer the chicken mixture to the pot with the broth mixture.
Cook on medium 45 minutes; reduce heat to low and
simmer another 45 minutes; ladle into bowls and top with
tortilla strips and cheese to serve.

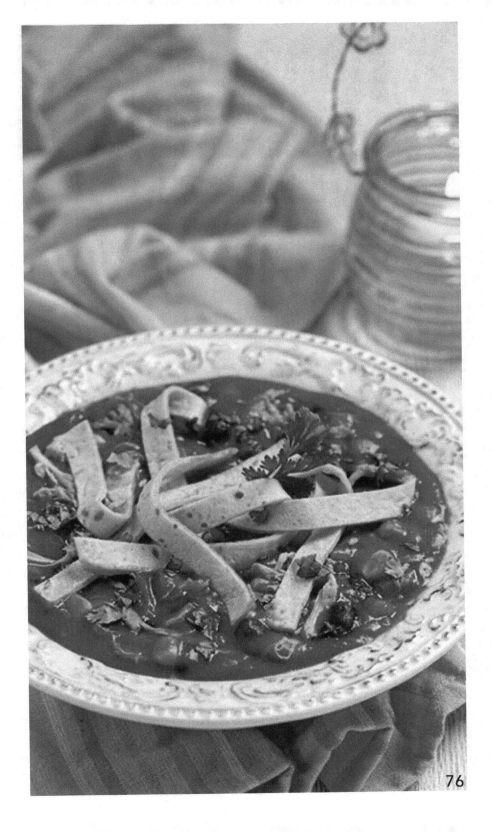

Green Bean Salad with Feta

Ingredients:

4 cups mixed baby salad greens

1/2 pound fresh green beans, trimmed, cooked al dente and cut in half

2 ounces feta cheese, crumbled | 2 tablespoons extra-virgin olive oil

1 tablespoon balsamic vinegar | 1 tablespoon orange juice

1/2 teaspoon fennel seeds Salt and pepper, to taste

1/3 cup dried cranberries (optional)

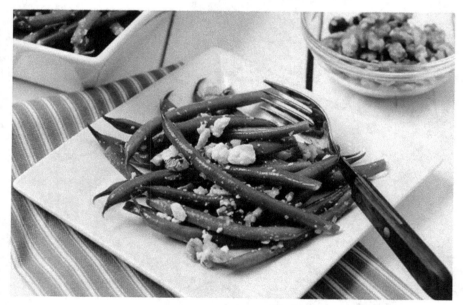

Directions:

In a medium-size bowl, combine greens, beans and cheese.
Add oil, vinegar, juice, fennel seeds, salt and pepper; toss.
Sprinkle with dried cranberries, if desired.

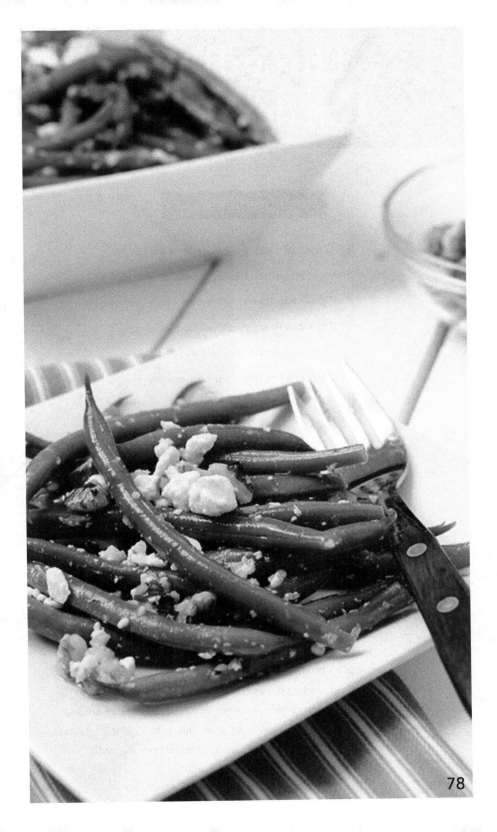

Three-Bean Garden Salad

1 (10 ounce) package frozen lima beans

1 (15 ounce) can kidney beans, rinsed and drained

1 (9 ounce) package frozen cut green beans, thawed

8 ounces fresh mushrooms, sliced

1 pint cherry tomatoes, halved

1/4 cup thinly sliced green onions

2/3 cup lemon juice

1/3 cup sugar

1/3 cup olive or vegetable oil

1 1/4 teaspoons salt

3/4 teaspoon Italian seasoning

1/2 teaspoon dried basil

1/2 teaspoon pepper

Directions:

Cook lima beans according to package directions.
Rinse in cold water; drain and place in a medium bowl.
Add kidney and green beans, mushrooms, tomatoes and onions.
Combine dressing ingredients. Pour over salad; mix gently to coat.
Cover and chill for at least 5 hours, stirring occasionally.

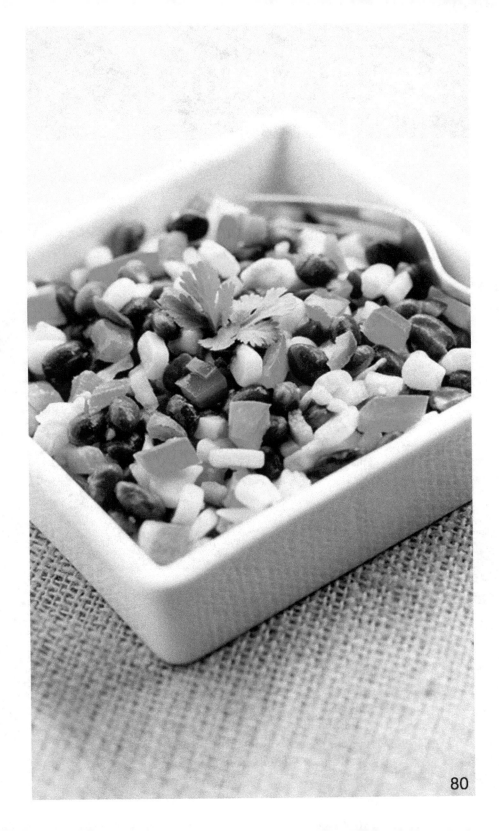

Pork BBQ

Ingredients:

1 pound cubed beef stew meat | 1 pound cubed pork loin

1 (10.75 ounce) can condensed tomato soup | 1/4 cup Worcestershire sauce

1/2 cup vinegar | 1 onion, diced

1 cup water

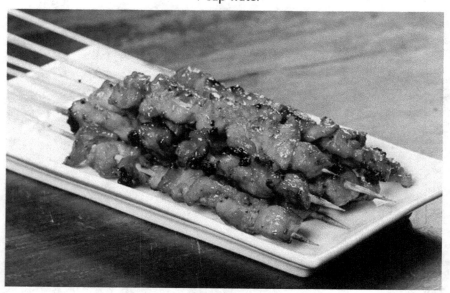

Directions:

Preheat oven to 350 degrees F (175 degrees C).

Combine together in a baking dish:

beef cubes, pork cubes, tomato soup, Worcestershire sauce,

vinegar, onion and water.

Bake in a preheated oven for 4 hours.

Add more water if liquid evaporates.

When done, remove from oven and shred with a

wooden fork or a potato masher.

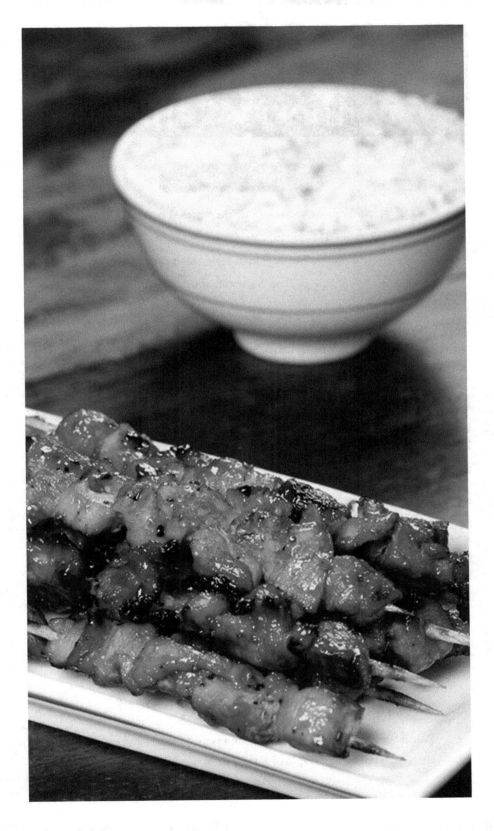

Easy Cranberry Chicken

6 skinless, boneless chicken breast halves

1 (16 ounce) can cranberry sauce

1 (8 ounce) bottle Ranch-style salad dressing

1/2 packet dry onion soup mix

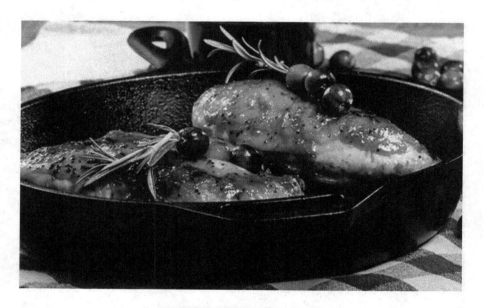

Directions:

Preheat oven to 350 degrees F (175 degrees C).

Place chicken breasts in a lightly greased 9x13 inch baking dish.

In a medium bowl, combine the cranberry sauce,

salad dressing and dry onion soup mix.

Blend together until well mixed, then pour mixture over chicken.

Bake at 350 degrees F (175 degrees C) for 1 hour

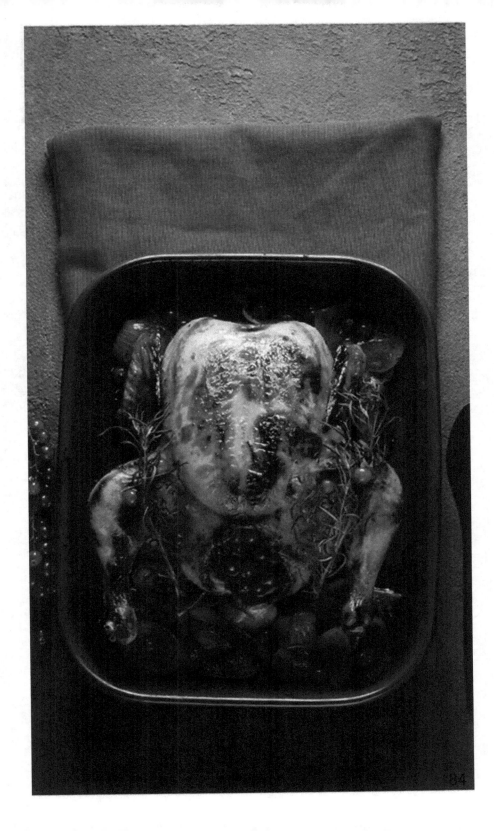

Hearty Pork N Beans

1 pound ground beef

1 medium green pepper, chopped

1 small onion, chopped

1 (1 pound) package smoked sausage,
halved lengthwise and thinly sliced

1 (16 ounce) can pork and beans, undrained

1 (15 ounce) can lima beans, rinsed and drained

1 (15 ounce) can pinto beans, rinsed and drained

1 cup ketchup

1/2 cup packed brown sugar

1 teaspoon salt

1/2 teaspoon garlic powder

1/4 teaspoon pepper

Directions:

In a skillet, cook beef, green pepper and onion over medium heat
until meat is no longer pink; drain.

In a slow cooker, combine the remaining ingredients.

Stir in beef mixture.

Cover and cook on high for 4-5 hours or until heated through.

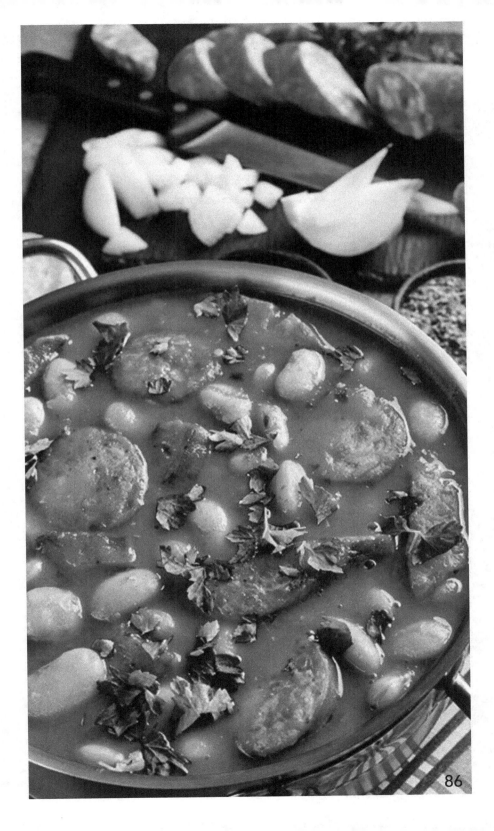

Becca's Barbequed Beans

Ingredients:

1 1/2 pounds lean ground beef

1/4 cup chopped onion

1/4 teaspoon ground black pepper

2/3 cup barbeque sauce

1/4 cup diced dill pickles

1 teaspoon Worcestershire sauce

2 (15 ounce) cans pork and beans

Directions:

Preheat oven to 350 degrees F (175 degrees C)

In a large skillet or saucepan, brown ground beef
and onion together with pepper, and drain well.

In a large casserole dish, combine beef mixture, barbeque sauce,
pickles, Worcestershire sauce, and pork and beans.

Cover with lid or foil, and bake in preheated oven
for 40 to 45 minutes, until hot and bubbly.

If you prefer, you can place the mixture in a slow cooker
at high heat, and simmer for 1 hour, or until hot.

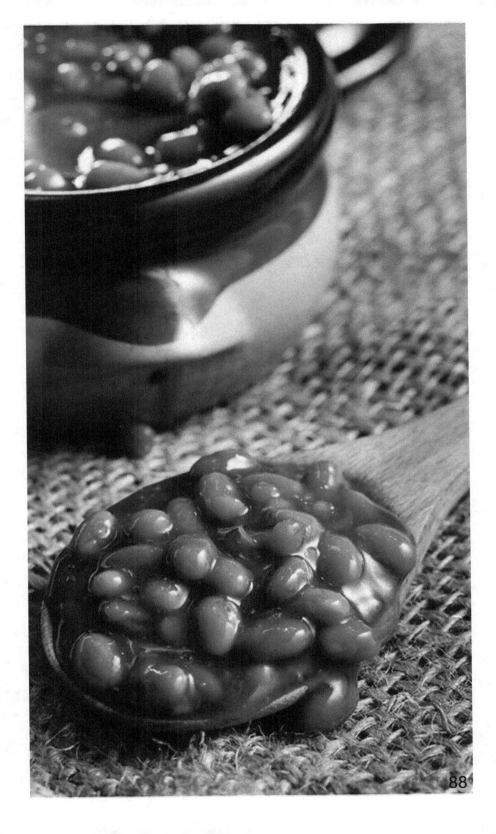

Mexican Pinto Beans

Ingredients:

1 pound dry pinto beans | 1/2 pound bacon

4 serrano peppers

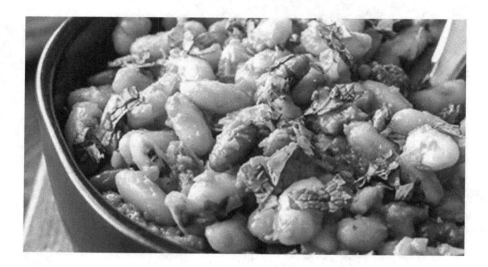

Directions:

Place the beans in a large pot with enough water to cover
by 3 to 4 inches, and bring to a boil.
Remove from heat, and let sit 1 hour.
Drain water. Pour in enough fresh water to cover beans
by 3 to 4 inches, and bring to a boil. Reduce heat, cover,
and simmer 1 hour.
Place bacon in a skillet, and cook over medium high heat
until evenly brown. Crumble bacon, and transfer,
along with grease, to the pot with the beans.
Continue to cook beans on low heat for 30 minutes.
Place the whole chile peppers into the pot,
and continue cooking beans 1 hour, or until tender.

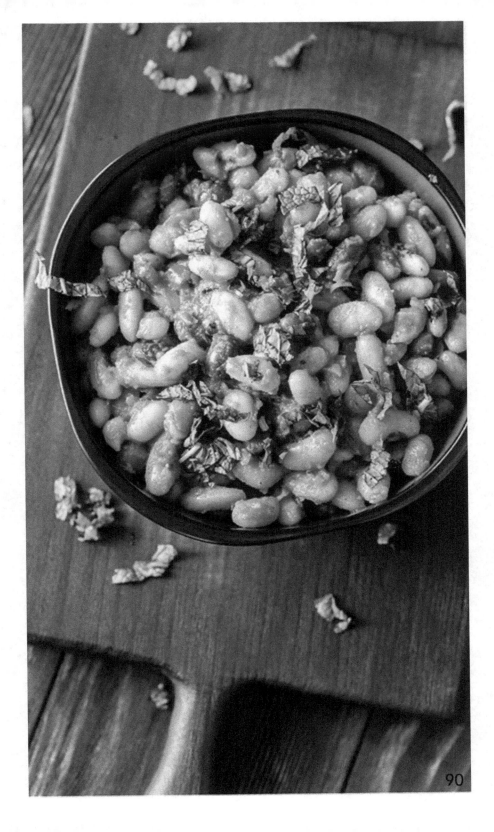

Italian Sausage Soup II

Ingredients:

2 tablespoons olive oil

1 pound Italian sausage, casings removed

1 1/2 cups chopped onion

1 1/2 cups sliced carrots

1 stalk celery with leaves, chopped

1 tablespoon chopped garlic

1 teaspoon dried basil

1 teaspoon dried rosemary

1/4 teaspoon dried crushed red pepper

1/4 teaspoon dried sage

1 (14.5 ounce) can canned diced tomatoes

5 cups chicken broth

1 (16 ounce) can kidney beans, drained

1 cup uncooked pasta shells

Directions:

Heat the oil in a large pot over medium-high heat.
Cook the sausage until evenly browned, and break into pieces.
Stir in the onions, carrots, celery, garlic, basil, rosemary,
red pepper, and sage.
Continue cooking 10 minutes, until vegetables are tender.
Mix in tomatoes, and cook until heated through.
Stir in the broth and beans. Bring to a boil.
Reduce heat to low, and simmer 20 minutes. Stir pasta into soup,
and continue cooking 10 minutes, or until pasta is al dente.

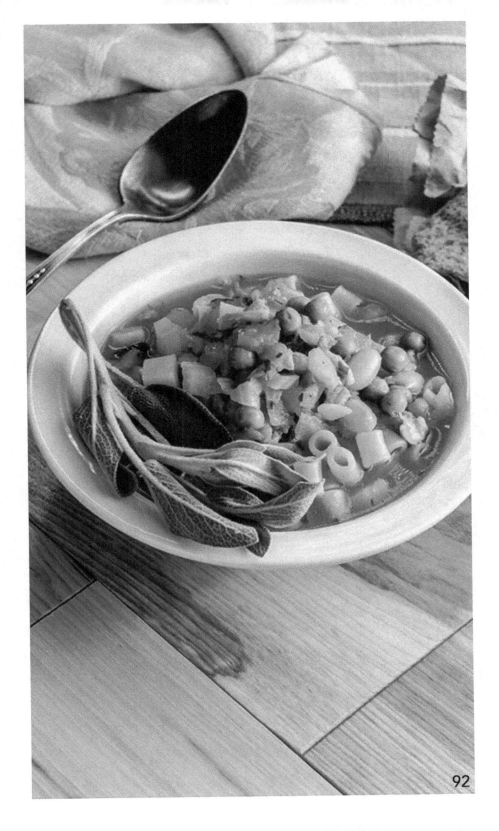

Vegetarian Kale Soup

2 tablespoons olive oil

1 yellow onion, chopped

2 tablespoons chopped garlic

1 bunch kale, stems removed and leaves chopped

8 cups water

6 cubes vegetable bouillon (such as Knorr)

1 (15 ounce) can diced tomatoes

6 white potatoes, peeled and cubed

2 (15 ounce) cans cannellini beans (drained if desired)

1 tablespoon Italian seasoning

2 tablespoons dried parsley

salt and pepper to taste

Directions:

Heat the olive oil in a large soup pot; cook the onion and garlic until soft.

Stir in the kale and cook until wilted, about 2 minutes.

Stir in the water, vegetable bouillon, tomatoes, potatoes, beans, Italian seasoning, and parsley.

Simmer soup on medium heat for 25 minutes, or until potatoes are cooked through.

Season with salt and pepper to taste.

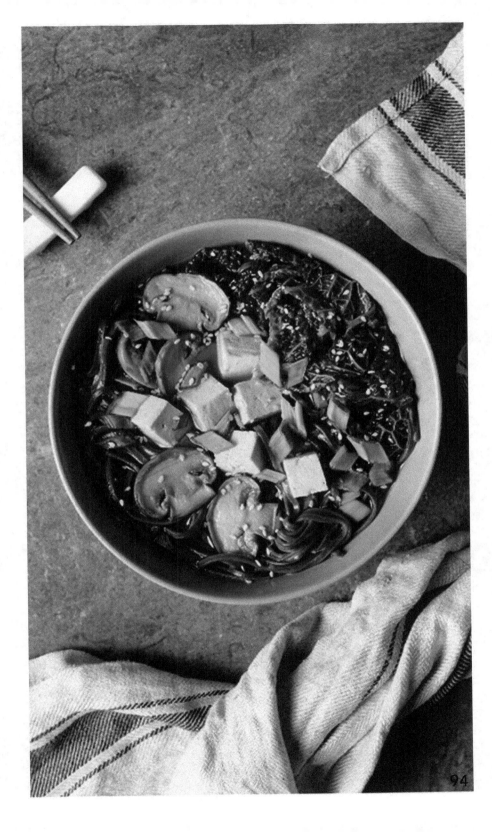

Tangy BBQ Ribs

Ingredients:

8 country style pork ribs | 1 cup honey

1 cup ketchup | 2 tablespoons molasses

1 (18 ounce) bottle barbeque sauce

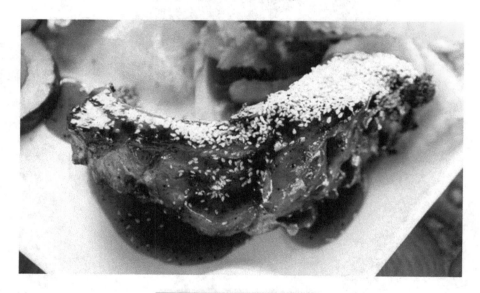

Directions:

Preheat grill for medium-high heat.
Lightly oil grill grate. Grill ribs for 12 minutes, turning once during cooking.
Transfer ribs to an 11x16 inch baking dish.
Preheat oven to 350 degrees F (175 degrees C).
In a large bowl, stir together the honey, ketchup, molasses,
and barbecue sauce.
Bake ribs, uncovered, for 1 hour.
Remove from the oven, and drain fat. Coat ribs with the honey sauce.
Continue baking for another 1 1/2 hours, or until ribs are tender.

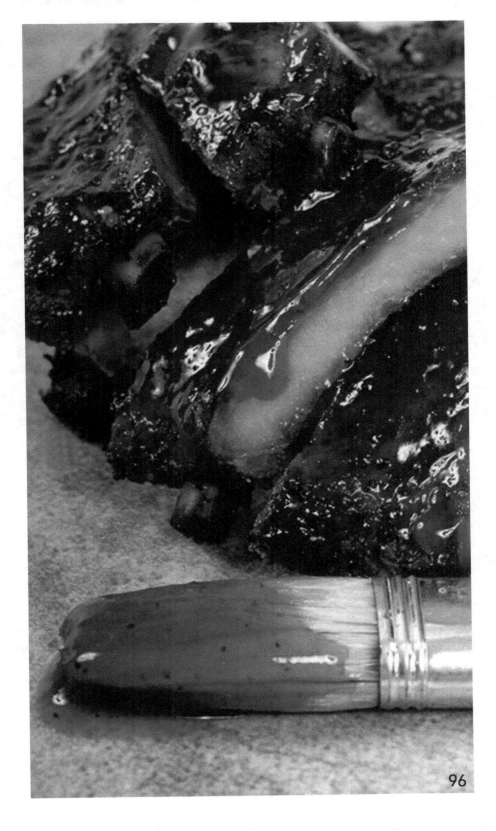

Three Bean and Artichoke Salad

Ingredients:

1 (15 ounce) can butter beans

1 (15 ounce) can kidney beans, drained and rinsed

1 (15 ounce) can green beans, drained

1 (14 ounce) can artichoke hearts, drained and quartered

4 tablespoons lemon juice | 4 tablespoons olive oil

2 tablespoons coarse grained prepared mustard | salt and pepper to taste

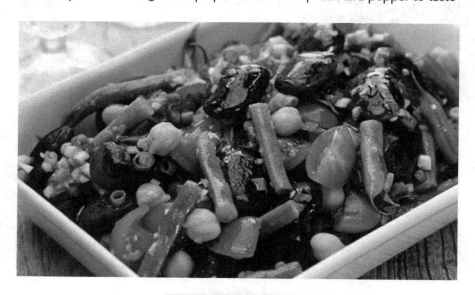

Directions:

In a medium bowl combine the butter beans,
kidney beans, green beans and artichoke hears.
In a small bowl, whisk together the lemon juice,
olive oil, mustard and salt and pepper to taste.
Toss with bean mixture and serve.

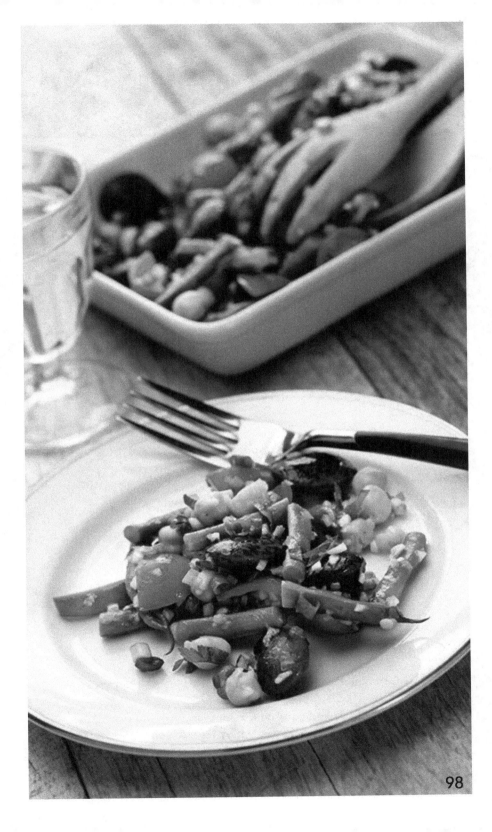

Beef Barley Lentil Soup

1 pound lean ground beef

medium onion, chopped

2 cups cubed red potatoes (1/4 inch pieces)

1 cup chopped celery

1 cup diced carrots

1 cup dry lentils, rinsed

1/2 cup medium pearl barley

8 cups water

2 teaspoons beef bouillon granules

1 teaspoon salt

1/2 teaspoon lemon-pepper seasoning

2 (14.5 ounce) cans stewed tomatoes

Directions:

In a nonstick skillet,
cook beef and onion over medium heat until
meat is no longer pink; drain.
Transfer to a 5-qt. slow cooker. Layer with the
potatoes, celery, carrots, lentils and barley.
Combine the water, bouillon, salt and lemon-pepper;
pour over vegetables.
Cover and cook on low for 6 hours or until
vegetables and barley are tender.
Add the tomatoes; cook 2 hours longer.

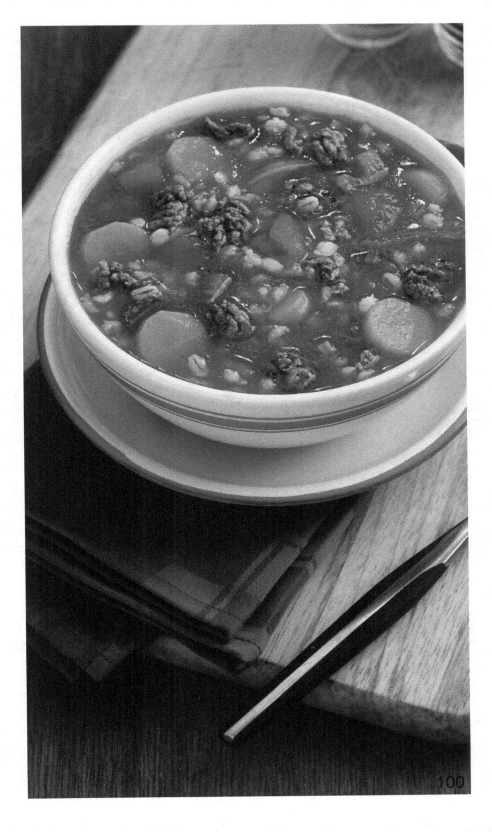

CPSIA information can be obtained
at www.ICGtesting.com
Printed in the USA
LVHW010524140521
687425LV00010B/726